Laboratory Quality
Management
QC ⇌ QA

Laboratory Quality Management
QC ⇌ QA

George S Cembrowski, MD, PhD

Director, Clinical Laboratories
Park Nicollet Medical Center

Clinical Assistant Professor
University of Minnesota
Minneapolis, MN

R Neill Carey, PhD

Clinical Chemist
Peninsula General Hospital

Clinical Associate Professor of Medical Technology
Salisbury State University
Salisbury, MD

ASCP Press
American Society of Clinical Pathologists · Chicago

Notice

Trade names and equipment and supplies described herein are included as suggestions only. In no way does their inclusion constitute an endorsement or preference by the American Society of Clinical Pathologists. The ASCP did not test the equipment, supplies, or procedures and, therefore, urges all readers to read and follow all manufacturers' instructions and package insert warnings concerning the proper and safe use of products.

Library of Congress Cataloging-in-Publication Data

Cembrowski, George S., 1949–
   Laboratory quality management.
   Includes bibliographies and index.
   1. Pathological laboratories—Quality control.

I. Carey, R. Neill, 1945–   . II. Title. [DNLM:
1. Laboratories—standards. 2. Pathology, Clinical—
standards. Quality Control. QY 23 C394L]
RB36.3.Q34C46 1989   616.07'5'0685   89-6729
ISBN 0-89189-277-X

Printed in the United States of America.

92   91   90   89   4   3   2   1

To Kay and Nancy

Contents

Figures

xiv

Tables

Foreword

Quality is a serious issue in health care today and this book provides a serious discussion of quality control practices in health care laboratories. George Cembrowski and Neill Carey provide the reader with both theory and practical applications of "state of the art" procedures in statistical quality control. Selected contributions from other authors broaden and extend the theory and practice of quality control.

Quality control is the foundation for developing quality management systems in health care laboratories. Although in widespread use since the 1960s, our understanding of QC procedures has tended to be qualitative. This book will help laboratory directors, managers, supervisors, and technologists move towards a more quantitative understanding of the performance capabilities of different quality control procedures. The quantitative nature of the materials makes the book an invaluable resource and reference.

Readers should understand that they will indeed have to study this book. It is not light reading, but it is essential reading and an essential reference for those who are involved in managing the quality of laboratory operations. And quality is going to be the key issue in laboratory testing in the 1990s, so this book deserves much study by laboratorians.

Most readers or students will want to study the first five chapters in sequence, beginning in Chapter 1 with the perspective on error prevention and error detection that has been learned in industrial quality management. Drawing on Juran's analysis of the quality control process, the authors define a framework for treating and assessing QC procedures in laboratory applications.

Chapter 2 covers basic statistical calculations in QC applications, as well as the elaborate calculations used in advanced techniques for trend analysis. The discussion of analytical errors and the treatment of components of variation provides additional background for understanding the next few chapters.

Chapters 3 and 4 describe reference sample QC procedures which use stable control materials as the samples to be analyzed. Chapter 3 deals with single-rule procedures, carefully defining the rules in use today and describing their performance characteristics in terms of probabilities of rejecting runs with differing amounts of errors. This quantitative treatment is applied to multi-rule procedures in Chapter 4 and extended to include some applications of predictive value theory to the QC testing situations.

Chapter 5 sets the stage for selecting and designing QC procedures based on quality requirements that reflect "medical usefulness." A thorough review is provided of the medical requirements recommended in the technical literature. The discussion of medical usefulness should be particularly useful to those analysts struggling to interpret current guidelines for application in designing QC procedures.

"Complicating Factors" is a good title for Chapter 6. It should prepare the reader for the most complicated materials and most complicated discussions that are to be encountered in the book. It contains a quantitative description of the effects of between run components of variation on the performance of QC procedures, something that we (George, Neill, Pierre and I) have been trying to figure out for years. It also contains some valuable information on the effects of data rounding that I have been waiting nearly ten years for George to put in writing. While much of this chapter is complicated, the recommendations, thankfully, are simple. An increased run component of variation will generally be harmful to the performance of QC procedures. Data rounding is potentially harmful for analytes whose QC range is reduced to less than 6 discrete intervals in the numerical scale of values observed for control measurements.

Many readers will probably want to read Chapter 8 next since it provides practical examples of the application of all the principles and theory. In fact, it may even be recommended prior to Chapter 6. The nuts and bolts of implementing QC procedures is described in detail, including examples that reduce all the theory to recommendations of what to do in specific situations. Much of Neill's "real world" experience shows here, and most laboratorians will find these examples very useful.

Chapter 7 on "patient data QC procedures" may actually tie with Chapter 6 for the most complicated material, as the authors show how the principles and theory developed for reference sample QC procedures also can be applied to patient data QC procedures. This chapter summarizes a whole body of work that George and a number of his colleagues have contributed over a decade or so. It is especially valuable when coupled with Chapter 9 which provides practical applications of these patient data procedures for quality control in hematology and coagulation laboratories. I am particularly delighted with the "quality control in hematology" chapter because it shows very clearly how the quantitative theory applies in areas other than clinical chemistry.

By this point in the book, readers will appreciate that QC can get pretty complicated and will be hoping for some help in reducing the difficulties by use of computers. Chapter 10 reviews the capabilities that can be expected in micro-processor controlled instrument systems, micro-computer application programs, and laboratory information systems.

In Chapter 11, the quantitative theory is extended to the area of external QC or proficiency testing. This extension is especially valuable in today's environment where more and more government regulations seem to be in the offing, with little understanding of what performance is to be expected by the proficiency testing schemes that are to be imposed. Chapter 12 concludes by reviewing the requirements being imposed by specific accrediting and regulatory agencies, and then returns to some broader issues in quality management in health care laboratories.

Having worked with George and Neill (and many of the other authors—Barry, Laessig, Ehrmeyer, Kurtycz), it is a pleasure to see how they have expanded and extended both the thinking and the applications of ideas that go back to some good times we enjoyed together at the University of Wisconsin several years ago. While they are colleagues instead of students, I have the same pride in their work and their accomplishments as if I were their teacher. I think it is the satisfaction of seeing the ideas developed and applied beyond my own visions and capabilities. That is the ultimate reward of being a teacher, and maybe I have played a little bit of that role with George and Neill ($p = 0.05$).

I can only add "tusen tak"—a thousand thanks—to George and Neill for providing us with this book, and another thousand thanks to Kay and Nancy for putting up with these two during the last three years while they were writing this.

James O. Westgard
University of Wisconsin
Madison, WI

Acknowledgments

We are indebted to many people for their support in producing *Laboratory Quality Management: QC and QA*. Specifically, we thank the ASCP Press for their support throughout the long process, especially Joshua Weikersheimer and Judy Hopping; Dr. Robert Rock for asking us to produce a book from our ASCP Workshop materials ("Improving Statistical Quality Control"); Ellen Lunetsky for her undaunted ability to design, program, and generate countless computer simulations and graphs; Dr. Pierre Douville for helpful discussions about statistical quality control and for fruitful joint research; Betsy Kind for her sensitive, capable editorial assistance; Dr. Robert Taylor for his continuing encouragement and helpful comments about the manuscript; Marjorie Wilson for her insight into hematology quality control; Gail Eckert for her insight into radioimmunoassay quality control; Bill Fore for his photographic talents; Paul Upham for his computer work; Drs. David Goodman and Leonard Jarett for providing a facilitating environment for much of GSC's research into laboratory quality practices. We thank our institutions and staffs for their support—Peninsula General Hospital (RNC) and Park Nicollet Medical Center and previously, the University of Pennsylvania (GSC).

We are grateful for the creativity and efforts of the coauthors of the four jointly written chapters and of the foreword: Patricia Barry and Dr. Pierre Douville (Chapter 6), Dr. Robert Hackney (Chapter 9), Dr. Daniel Kui·iycz (Chapter 10), Drs. Sharon Ehrmeyer and Ronald Laessig (Chapter 11), and Dr. James Westgard (Foreword).

We especially thank two of our teachers: Dr. Cliff Toren, our graduate advisor, for showing us the potential applications of analytical chemistry in the clinical laboratory, and Dr. James Westgard, for inspiring us, and continually sharing his ideas and observations. Jim introduced us to the concepts of quality management and taught us the value of investigating and optimizing routine laboratory practices. Through his example of teaching, he showed us the importance of popularizing our findings.

Most of all, we thank our wives, Kay and Nancy, for their support and understanding during this three-year project.

Laboratory Quality Management
QC ⇌ QA

CHAPTER ONE

Quality Control of the Testing Process

THE "QUALITY REVOLUTION"

During the 1970s and early 1980s, foreign manufacturers increased their market share worldwide at the expense of the American manufacturing industry. While lower labor costs, unfair trade practices, and restrictive tariffs were initially invoked to explain the new competitive advantage, subsequent analysis established the superior quality of the foreign manufactured product to be the primary competitive force. Through studies of successful American and foreign corporations, American companies began to relearn the tenet of America's quality control leaders: improvement of a product's quality can markedly decrease the effort and expense necessary to produce, market, and maintain that product. In this decade, the focus of management has shifted from programs which emphasize short-term costs to programs which emphasize product quality.

This change in management focus has begun to revitalize the American manufacturing industry. Many of the concepts described in the recent industrial quality management literature[1-6] are directly applicable to the health care area. Quality in the clinical laboratory testing process has long been an important issue, and most laboratorians are already very quality conscious. However, over the last decade, many hospital and laboratory administrators have had to relearn the lessons of the American manufacturer: the cost of production can be very expensive when there is insufficient emphasis on quality.

QUALITY CHARACTERISTICS, QUALITY REQUIREMENTS, AND QUALITY CONTROL

In order to fully appreciate the impact of quality in the clinical laboratory, the meaning of *quality* in laboratory testing must be under-

1

stood. Juran[5] defined quality as "fitness for use." Crosby[1] has defined quality as "conformance to requirements." Whose uses or requirements are being considered? In business, they are usually the customer's. In today's health care environment, the definition of the customer is complex. The customer can be the health care provider (clinician), the health care purchaser (patient or corporation), or the ultimate recipient of the health care, the patient. The requirements of each of these customers can diverge, even in the provision of a single laboratory test. For example, the clinician usually requires speed and accuracy in analysis and reporting, the health care purchaser requires inexpensive but highly diagnostic tests, and the patient requires the security that the laboratory test is being performed in the best possible manner. The indicators of a test's quality, including turnaround time, accuracy, cost, and diagnostic effectiveness, are called *quality characteristics*. Specifications or requirements can be set for each of these quality characteristics and are referred to as *quality specifications* or *quality requirements*. For example, a maximum turnaround time can be set for specimen testing, eg, 20 minutes for the analysis of an arterial specimen for blood gases; this turnaround time of 20 minutes would comprise a quality specification for the quality characteristic turnaround time.

Laboratory testing is complex. After a clinician orders a laboratory test, a series of events occurs, beginning with the transcription of the order and ending with receipt of the test result by the clinician (Figure 1-1). After a test is ordered, a specimen is collected from the patient, labeled, and transported to the laboratory. The specimen is prepared and analyzed, and the test results are reported to the clinician who then interprets the test results and treats the patient accordingly. A problem in any of the steps can cause errors or delays in the result and cause the result to be useless.

Each step of the process has its own quality characteristics whose quality requirements must be achieved so that the laboratory test will be fit for use. Another quality characteristic in the test ordering stage is the clarity of communications among the clinician, the ward clerk or nurse, and the person collecting and labeling the specimen. The patient's identity, the laboratory tests being ordered, and the patient's preparation (fasting, post-transfusion, etc) must be clearly indicated. Miscommunication can result in obtaining the specimen from the wrong patient, performing the wrong test, or obtaining misleading test results because of inappropriate patient preparation. In the sample preparation step, timeliness, preservation of specimen integrity, and correct specimen identification are important quality characteristics.

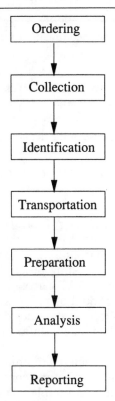

Figure 1–1 Steps in the medical laboratory testing process.

Each step must be controlled so that the final product, the result of the laboratory test, is fit for use. The quality control process consists of observing the actual performance, comparing the performance with a standard for performance, and then taking action if the observed performance is significantly different from the standard. Juran describes this control process as a *feedback loop* consisting of the sequence of steps[5] listed in Table 1–1.

Some illustrations help demonstrate this process. One of the most important quality characteristics of the entire testing process is timeliness. The within laboratory turnaround times for STAT glucose testing are monitored at Peninsula General Hospital. The quality specification (or performance standard) set in conjunction with the Emergency Department Medical Staff defined the within laboratory turnaround time for STAT glucose tests as less than 40 minutes for 90% of the specimens

Table 1-1 Steps in the control process.

1. Choose what is to be controlled (quality characteristic).
2. Choose a unit of measurement.
3. Set a standard for the quality characteristic.
4. Choose a sensing device which can measure the quality characteristic in terms of the unit of measurement.
5. Measure the actual performance.
6. Interpret the difference between the actual quality and the standard.
7. Take action (if any) on the difference.

Modified with permission. From Juran JM, Gryna FM: Quality planning and analysis. McGraw-Hill, New York, 1980, pp 1-3.

tested. The "sensing device" (see Table 1-1) is the laboratory information system which provides a time stamp at each stage of the testing process. Whenever the turnaround times fail to meet the specification, the specimen handling and testing processes are investigated for the cause. In this example, each STAT glucose specimen's turnaround time is monitored; thus there should be no question of whether the quality specification is being met, and computer detection of failure to meet specification is certain. The report states the percentage of specimens which met the requirement.

Usually, the quality characteristic cannot be monitored so directly or so absolutely. As mentioned before, correct specimen identification in the sample preparation and sample analysis steps constitutes such a quality characteristic (ie, lack of specimen mixups). The quality specification requires that no result be reported from a specimen suspected of being misidentified. One of the most common sensing devices for misidentification is the "delta check" in which the current test results are compared to the patient's previous results. Limits for the maximum amount of disagreement are set in terms of result units for each test performed. Specimens with a disagreement exceeding these limits for any test are investigated, and appropriate corrective actions are taken if misidentification is confirmed (see Chapter 7). In this example the sensing device does not monitor specimen identification directly, but rather checks for unusually large disagreements between serial patient results. Unfortunately, the monitoring of delta checks is inexact. It cannot detect all mixups, furthermore, mixups may be signaled when none have occurred.

ERROR PREVENTION *v* ERROR DETECTION

These examples demonstrate that assuring quality in laboratory medicine requires both error prevention and error detection. *Error*

4

prevention involves developing a laboratory process inherently capable of meeting the quality specifications required for medical usefulness. *Error detection* involves examination of the process for the presence of error. Error detection is the monitoring activity of quality control. If an error is detected by monitoring and cannot be tolerated, the patient sample(s) must be recollected and/or reanalyzed following appropriate corrective action. Monitoring of the laboratory process for purposes of error detection is essential, but it cannot detect every error; thus problems associated with a particular specimen or general problems with the analytical process may go undetected.

Thus, error prevention is enhanced in patient specimen identification by development and implementation of specimen handling procedures which minimize opportunities for error to occur, careful training of personnel, sufficient staffing, and watchful supervision. Error prevention is an activity which determines the inherent quality of the testing process. A process which inherently produces many errors (relative to the quality specification) requires much more sensitive error detection to maintain an acceptable rate of errors than a process which produces few errors. Although the delta checking referred to in the above example is a useful error detection tool for detecting patient specimen mixups, its performance for error detection is rather weak, and many specimen errors could occur without detection (see Chapter 7). Thus the phlebotomy and sample preparation stages of the testing process require a vigorous program of error prevention in order to meet quality requirements.

Traditionally, clinical laboratory quality control practices have focused on error detection; actually a coordinated combination of error prevention and error detection is required.

QUALITY ASSURANCE AND QUALITY CONTROL

Two terms, *quality control* and *quality assurance,* are used to refer to the control of the testing process to insure that the test results meet their quality requirements. The terms quality control and quality assurance have overlapping definitions, and are frequently used interchangeably, even by experts. Attempts to completely differentiate these terms often result in tedious definitions. Quality control includes establishing specifications for each quality characteristic of the testing process, assessing the procedures used in the testing process to determine conformance to these specifications, and taking any necessary corrective actions to bring them into conformance.[7-9] Quality assurance is more expansive and not only encompasses the quality control

5

Table 1–2 Comparison of quality control to quality assurance practices.

Identifying Characteristics	Quality Control	Quality Assurance
Primary concern	control	coordination
View of quality	a problem to be solved	a problem to be solved but one that is attacked proactively
Emphasis	product uniformity with reduced inspection	the entire production chain, from design to market, and the contribution of all functional groups, especially designers, to preventing quality failures
Methods	statistical tools and techniques	programs and systems
Role of quality professionals	trouble-shooting and the application of statistical methods	quality measurement, quality planning, and program design
Who has responsibility for quality	the manufacturing and engineering department	all departments, although top management is only peripherally involved in designing, planning, and executing quality policies
Orientation and approach	"controls in" quality	"builds in" quality

Reproduced with permission. From Garvin DA: Managing quality: the strategic and competitive edge. Free Press, New York, 1983, p 37.

of the testing process, but also involves monitoring and control of the ultimate outcomes of the testing process, including patient morbidity, patient satisfaction, and financial costs attributable to the laboratory. Garvin's comparison of quality control practices to quality assurance practices is shown in Table 1–2. Quality assurance topics are specifically covered in more detail in Chapter 12.

QUALITY CHARACTERISTICS OF THE ANALYTICAL STAGE

The quality characteristics of the analytical stage are numerous. Peters and Westgard[10] have divided them into practicality and reliability characteristics. These characteristics, listed in Table 1–3, should be considered whenever a new analytical method or instrument is being

Table 1-3 Quality characteristics of the analytical process.

Practicality characteristics:
  specimen handling requirements
  minimum sample size
  throughput (capacity)
  personnel skill
  cost per test
  method of standardization
  methods of quality control
  space needs (including reagent storage)
  turnaround time including that for "stat" specimens
  precautions and procedures required for safety

Reliability characteristics:
  precision
  accuracy
  analytical sensitivity
  analytical specificity
  recovery
  interference
  blank readings
  linear range
  sample interaction
  reagent stability

Modified with permission. From Peters T, Westgard JO: Evaluation of methods. In: Tietz NW, ed: Textbook of clinical chemistry. Saunders, Philadelphia, 1986, pp 410-411.

selected. The maximum quality achievable is highly method-dependent and fixed once the method is selected. Thus, selection and evaluation of analytical methods are important error prevention activities. If the method is not inherently capable of providing the required quality (weak error prevention), no amount of error detection activity can make its performance acceptable.

Traditionally, the laboratorian has equated the term quality control to the quality control of the analytical stage of the laboratory testing process. Here, *precision* and *accuracy* are the quality characteristics which must be controlled within medically defined quality specifications. In the control process, the unit of quality measurement is the unit of the analyte. The sensing device often consists of reference samples (the formal name for "controls") which are analyzed with each group of patient specimens. The performance standard consists of statistically derived *control limits* within which reference sample results are acceptable. If the reference sample results fall outside the control limits, the analytical method may be at fault and should be investigated.

If necessary, the analytical process is corrected and the patient and reference samples are reanalyzed. As will be seen in later chapters, the control limits for a quality control procedure are usually statistically derived parameters which describe the inherent analytical performance of the method. Unless the control limits (performance standard) for the quality control procedure have been derived with consideration of both the inherent errors of the method *and* the quality specification for accuracy and precision, the method could be "in control," yet the results could lack the medically required accuracy and precision.

The importance of error prevention in providing quality laboratory results can be demonstrated further by considering the analysis of samples with a method that is capable of precision and accuracy which exceed the precision and accuracy required for medical use. The method will produce few results whose errors exceed the medical specification. Thus, when the method is subjected to quality control to detect the presence of increased error and prevent reporting results when the method's performance degrades, an acceptably low rate of errors should occur in the reported patient results. As was pointed out earlier, the choice of method limits the precision and accuracy attainable during routine operation. This concept is discussed further in Chapters 5 and 8.

INTERNAL *v* EXTERNAL QUALITY CONTROL

Quality control of the measurement stage may be divided into 2 major practices, *internal* quality control and *external* quality control. In internal quality control, the source of specimens is the same laboratory which does the testing. These specimens may be reference samples or patient specimens. There is little or no delay in the internal quality control feedback loop consisting of measurement, interpreting the difference between the actual performance and the performance standard, and taking action. Internal quality control practices are thus used for immediate decisions to accept or reject the results of tests on a group of patient specimens.

In external quality control, an external source distributes specimens as "unknowns" to multiple participating laboratories. Upon receipt, the laboratories analyze the specimens and return the analytical results to the testing center. The testing center then summarizes the data for the unknowns and returns a statistical summary to each participating laboratory. There is a delay between analysis and receipt of the statistical summary; this delay can be as long as 3 months. While it is essential for the laboratory with outlying results to identify and correct any sources of error, the delay often obscures the origin of the error. External quality control is further discussed in Chapter 11.

THE COST OF QUALITY

Given the emphasis laboratorians place on quality, it should not be surprising that an average of approximately 25% of the consumable costs of clinical laboratories are for quality control.[11] For some assays, the quality control consumables can amount to 50% of the cost of the testing effort,[12] although in very large, efficient laboratories, quality control costs have been reduced to as low as 10% of the consumable costs.[13] Quality control as practiced in the clinical laboratory is expensive in terms of time, consumable materials, and excess laboratory testing. Its benefits may not be immediately obvious, and the improvement in quality brought about by an increase in quality control activity has been hard to quantify.

The true cost of quality can be assessed from the perspective of overall patient care. Quality control reduces the frequency of erroneous test results. The costs of erroneous results include those of repeat testing, duplicate testing, and difficult-to-document costs including prolonged patient stays, poor patient outcomes, and malpractice lawsuits. In this context, quality control is actually a cost cutting tool. Westgard and Barry have judiciously summarized the philosophy that quality management programs can actually save money when the hidden cost of erroneous laboratory testing results is considered.[6]

APPLICATION OF QUALITY CONTROL THEORY IN LABORATORY MEDICINE

The theoretical basis of laboratory quality control has advanced dramatically in the past 15 years. If the quality requirements for an analyte are defined, and the analytical errors of the method are characterized, the error detection performance required of the quality control system can be calculated in order to maintain analytical errors within the quality specification. The effect of the selected quality control procedures on the quality of the test results can be predicted. The error detection performance of quality control procedures has been explored and can now be better optimized in actual practice. Compared to previously practiced quality control procedures, modern procedures are more cost effective and are better able to distinguish between real errors and problem-free operation.

9

REFERENCES

1. Crosby PB: Quality is free. McGraw-Hill, New York, 1979.
2. Waterman RH: The renewal factor. Bantam, New York, 1987.
3. Townsend PL: Commit to quality. John Wiley, New York, 1986.
4. Harrington HJ: The improvement process. McGraw-Hill, New York, 1987.
5. Juran JM, Gryna FM: Quality planning and analysis. McGraw-Hill, New York, 1980.
6. Westgard JO, Barry PL: Cost-effective quality control: managing the quality and productivity of analytical processes. AACC Press, Washington, DC, 1986.
7. Subcommittee on analytical goals in clinical chemistry, World Association of Societies of Pathology, Ciba Foundation, London, April 25–28, 1978: Analytical goals in clinical chemistry: their relationship to medical care. Am J Clin Pathol 71:624-630, 1979.
8. Taylor JK: Quality assurance of chemical measurements. Lewis, Chelsea, Michigan, 1987.
9. Anon: Quality assurance in the laboratory. Can J Med Technol 46(2):69-70, 1984.
10. Peters T, Westgard JO: Evaluation of methods. In: Tietz NW, ed: Textbook of clinical chemistry. Saunders, Philadelphia, 1986, pp 410-411.
11. Tydeman J, Morrison JI, Cassidy PA, Hardwick DF, Chase WH: Analyzing the factors contributing to raising laboratory costs. Working paper, p 91, Institute for the Future, Palo Alto, California 1980.
12. Bercz JP: Cost effectiveness of esoteric testing. Lab Management 13:32-34, 1975.
13. O'Sullivan MB, Pfaff KJ, Dunemann SE, Scheffel JG: Group lab: key to economic survival. Group Practice Journal 35(2):4-12, 1986.

CHAPTER TWO

Statistical Background: Introduction to Reference Sample Quality Control

Quality control procedures were originally derived from simple population statistics. Recently formulated quality control theory, too, is a logical extension of these same statistics. The understanding of quality control thus requires some familiarity with basic population statistics. This chapter presents only the minimum background in order to understand quality control procedures; the interested reader is encouraged to consult standard sources[1,2,3] for further information.

STATISTICAL DESCRIPTIONS OF POPULATIONS

Mean, Standard Deviation, z-Score, Coefficient of Variation

Laboratory measurement is inexact. When a specimen is analyzed repetitively under identical conditions (same analyst using the same equipment and reagents), a series of nonidentical results is obtained. These nonidentical values arise from the random variation that is inherent in all measurement processes. When many results are obtained from the repeated analysis of a single stable specimen by a stable method, their frequency distribution will approximate a normal or gaussian distribution. Figure 2–1 shows a frequency histogram of glucose results obtained by analyzing such a stable sample on many occasions. Results in the center of the distribution occur more frequently than those farther away. Usually the distribution of results approximates a gaussian distribution, and the value at the center of the distribution is the arithmetic mean. The mean is a measure of central tendency and is the simple average of all results. The mean is calculated by dividing the sum of all results by the number of results, as in

11

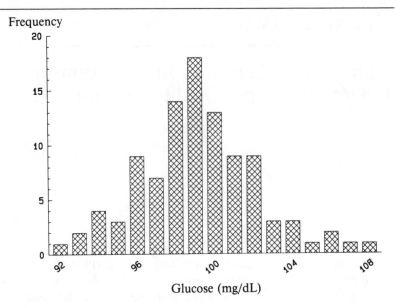

Figure 2-1   Frequency histogram of glucose control data, $\bar{x}$ = 100.0, s = 3.0 mg/dL.

Equation 2-1. The mean of the glucose values of Figure 2-1 is 100.0 mg/dL.

$$\bar{x} = \frac{\Sigma \bar{x}_i}{N},$$ Eq. 2-1

where
$\bar{x}$ = mean of all x_i,
N   = number of values,
x_i = ith value,
Σx_i = sum of all x_i.

Another measure of central tendency is the median. It is determined by first arranging the results in order of increasing or decreasing size. The median is the middle result; half of the results are higher than the median, and half are lower. If the number of results is even, the median is derived by summing the 2 innermost observations and dividing by 2. The median of the glucose results of Figure 2-1 is 100 mg/dL. For gaussian distributions, the values of the mean and median should be almost equal.

12

The dispersion of gaussian data about their mean can be expressed by the standard deviation s, which is calculated according to Equation 2–2.

$$s = \sqrt{\frac{\Sigma(x_i - \bar{x})^2}{N - 1}}.$$

Eq. 2–2

Figure 2–2 illustrates how the distribution of gaussian data around their mean is described by the standard deviation. Approximately two thirds of the results, 68.3%, are located within the interval bounded by the $\bar{x} \pm 1.0s$ lines; 95.5% are within the $\bar{x} \pm 2.0s$ lines, and 99.7% are within the $\bar{x} \pm 3.0s$ lines. These intervals containing specific fractions of the population correspond to specific *confidence intervals*. Thus, the $\bar{x} \pm 2s$ interval is the 95.5% confidence interval. There is approximately a 95.5% probability that any given result will fall within the $\bar{x} \pm 2s$ lines. Conversely, there is a 4.5% chance that a result will fall outside these lines. For the $\bar{x} \pm 3s$ interval, there is approximately a 99.7% probability that a result will be inside the limits, and only a 0.3% chance that a result will be outside the limits. Constructing confidence limits in this manner assumes that the data have a gaussian distribution, and that sufficient data have been obtained for the mean and standard deviation to be known accurately. If a population has a gaussian distribution, only the mean and standard deviation are necessary to describe the population. According to Taylor, quality control data may be assumed to be normally distributed for "all practical purposes."[4] Virtually all quality control procedures used in the clinical laboratory assume a gaussian distribution. Causes of deviations from a gaussian distribution include: outliers, shifts, nonrandom variation, and instability of the analytic method.[4]

The *variance* is the standard deviation squared (s^2). The variance is used in many statistical calculations; examples are shown later in this chapter.

The standard deviation is sometimes presented as a percentage relative to the mean, as the *coefficient of variation* (CV).

$$CV(\%) = 100\,\frac{s}{\bar{x}}.$$

Eq. 2–3

The CV, also known as the relative standard deviation, is a unitless number which simplifies the comparison of standard deviations of test results expressed at different concentrations or in different units. Calculations of mean, variance, standard deviation, and coefficient of variation are illustrated in Example 2–1.

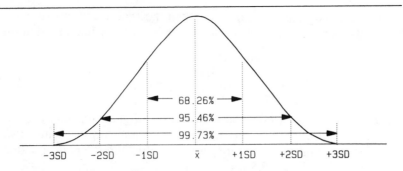

Figure 2-2   Gaussian distribution. SD = standard deviation.

If duplicate measurements are available on a set of specimens, the *standard deviation of the duplicates* can be calculated from the differences of each pair. This measure of dispersion is attractive because it is obtained from actual patient specimens rather than control materials (more about control materials in Chapters 6 and 8). The calculation is made according to Equation 2-4:

$$s = \sqrt{\frac{\Sigma(x_{i1} - x_{i2})^2}{2N}},$$ Eq. 2-4

where
s   = standard deviation of duplicates,
x_{i1} = first duplicate result for sample x_i,
x_{i2} = second duplicate result for sample x_i,
N   = number of samples tested in duplicate.

The mean and standard deviation describe the distribution of a set of results. On occasion, it is useful to represent the position of a single result within the distribution. The position of the result may be expressed by the number of standard deviations it differs from the mean. This difference from the mean, termed the *z-score* or SDI (standard deviation index), is calculated by Equation 2-5, where z is the z-score:

$$z = \frac{x_i - \bar{x}}{s}.$$ Eq. 2-5

The z-score expresses a result's position in the distribution independent of concentration.

14

EXAMPLE 2–1 Calculation of population statistics.

When plasma theophylline measurements were made repeatedly on a specimen from a 13-year-old male who had symptoms of theophylline toxicity, the following results (in mg/L) were obtained: 23, 26, 24, 22, 24, 23, 21, 26, 25, 24, 22, 23, 25, 23, 22, 24, 23, 25, 24, 22.

Calculate the mean, variance, standard deviation, and coefficient of variation of these replicates.

$$\text{mean, } \bar{x} = \frac{\Sigma x_i}{N} = \frac{471}{20} = 23.55 \text{ mg/L,}$$

$$\text{variance, } s^2 = \frac{\Sigma(x_i - \bar{x})^2}{N - 1}.$$

An alternative formula which simplifies calculation of the variance is

$$\text{variance, } s^2 = \frac{N\Sigma x_i^2 - (\Sigma x_i)^2}{N(N - 1)},$$

$$\text{standard deviation} = s.$$

The table below demonstrates both methods of calculation.

x_i	x_i^2	$(x_i - \bar{x})$	$(x_i - \bar{x})^2$
23	529	0.55	0.3025
26	676	2.45	6.0025
24	576	0.45	0.2025
22	484	1.55	2.4025
24	576	0.45	0.2025
23	529	0.55	0.3025
21	441	2.55	6.5025
26	676	2.45	6.0025
25	625	1.45	2.1025
24	576	0.45	0.2025
22	484	1.55	2.4025
23	529	0.55	0.3025
25	625	1.45	2.1025
23	529	0.55	0.3025
22	484	1.55	2.4025
24	576	0.45	0.2025
23	529	0.55	0.3025
25	625	1.45	2.1025
24	576	0.45	0.2025
22	484	1.55	2.4025
471	11,129	N/A	36.9500

$$\bar{x} = \frac{\Sigma x_i}{N} = \frac{471}{20} = 23.55 \text{ mg/L,}$$

$$s^2 = \frac{\Sigma(x_i - \bar{x})^2}{N - 1} = \frac{36.95}{19} = 1.9447, \text{ or}$$

$$s^2 = \frac{N\Sigma x_i^2 - (\Sigma x_i)^2}{N(N - 1)} = \frac{20(11,129) - 4712}{20(19)} = 1.9447.$$

$$s = 1.39 \text{ mg/L,}$$

$$CV = \frac{100 \text{ s}}{\bar{x}} = \frac{100(1.39)}{23.55} = 5.90\%.$$

Confidence Intervals for Means

The uncertainty of single measurements can be reduced by performing multiple measurements, pooling the data and calculating a mean. The *standard deviation of the mean*, usually referred to as the standard error of the mean (SEM), is given by Equation 2–6.:

$$SEM = \frac{s}{\sqrt{N}}. \qquad \text{Eq. 2–6}$$

If groups of control results are averaged, the distribution of the means of the individual groups around the grand mean (average of the averages) will be described by the grand mean and the SEM. Confidence limits for the mean are set about the grand mean using SEM instead of s. Thus, the 99% confidence limits for a mean would be $\bar{x} \pm 2.58$ SEM. As more and more observations are incorporated in the mean, the SEM will approach 0, and there will be little uncertainty about the location of the mean.

REFERENCE SAMPLE QUALITY CONTROL

The confidence limits for groups of observations constitute the foundation of statistical quality control as it is currently practiced in most laboratories. These confidence limits are generated from the replicate analysis of a stable specimen, usually commercially available *control material* (or control product). For chemistry, the control material is most often a lyophilized pool of many specimens, although frozen aliquots of a pool are often used. For hematology, the control material is usually a solution of chemically stabilized red and white cells. The most important characteristics of a control material are its stability and its physical similarity to a real patient sample. If a control material is not stable, its instability will artefactually increase the apparent random variation of the analytical method. If its physical characteristics vary from those of a patient specimen, its analytical behavior may be significantly different from that of a patient specimen. During testing, the control material should be treated exactly like a patient sample.

The confidence limits used for control materials in routine testing are termed *control limits*. To determine control limits, the control material is repetitively analyzed during a period when the analytical method is thought to be in stable operation. The mean and standard deviation are calculated from the replicate determinations and are used to derive control limits. Results obtained from subsequent analyses of the control material are interpreted by reference to these control limits characterizing stable operation. This quality control system is known as reference sample quality control.

Because control results outside the $\bar{x} \pm 3s$ interval occur infrequently when the method is stable (3 out of 1000 occasions), many laboratories use the $\bar{x} \pm 3s$ limits as control limits. The $\bar{x} \pm 3s$ control limits for the glucose values of Figure 2–1 would be 100 mg/dL $\pm$ (3 $\times$ 3 mg/dL) or 91 to 109 mg/dL. When control results outside these limits are obtained, they indicate that the method is possibly operating in a manner different from when the original control results were obtained, and therefore indicate the likelihood of increased analytical error. Other frequently employed control limits include $\bar{x} \pm 1.96s$, corresponding to the 95% confidence interval, $\bar{x} \pm 2s$, corresponding to the 95.5% confidence interval, and $\bar{x} \pm 2.58s$, corresponding to the 99% confidence limits. When control results are distributed as expected within the above confidence limits, the analytical process is assumed to be in a state of statistical control or "in control." Whenever control results beyond the chosen limits are obtained, an error condition is implied, and investigation and/or corrective action is required.

INHERENT ANALYTICAL VARIATION

Every analytical method demonstrates some variation; this variation can be decreased to a minimum level, but can never be completely eliminated. The inherent analytical variation has many causes, some of which are related solely to the analytical method, some to the reagents and controls, and some to the laboratory setting in which the method is operated. These components of inherent variation are usually categorized by the period over which they operate, short term and long term. Sources of variation, as categorized by Brauer and Rand,[5] are summarized in Table 2–1.

Table 2-1   Sources of analytical variation.

Within Run
  Sample and/or reagent metering variation
  Sample evaporation
  Photometric variation
  Incubation temperature variation
  Electronic drift

Run to Run
  Random calibration error if each run separately calibrated
  Calibrator and/or control fluid deterioration after reconstitution
  Operator-to-operator variation

Day to Day
  Control or calibrator vial-to-vial variation
  Reconstitution variation
  Random calibration error if 1 calibration per day

Week to Week
  Calibrator and/or control fluid deterioration
  Uncalibratable reagent change
  Uncalibratable analyzer response change caused by change in operating
    environment

Modified with permission. From Brauer and Rand: In: Quality assurance in health care: A critical appraisal of clinical chemistry. Rand RN, Eilers RJ, Lawson NS, Broughton A, eds. American Association for Clinical Chemistry 1980, p 212.

Short-Term (within Run) Variation

Short-term variation generally refers to the variation observed in results accumulated *within 1 calibration and over a short time period* (one half day or less). Short-term variation is defined as *within run* variation. Traditionally, an analytical run has consisted of calibrator, control, and patient specimens, analyzed as a batch, without interruption.[6] The within-run standard deviation is abbreviated s_w, with "w" standing for *within run*. Short-term variation is often estimated from the standard deviation of patient or control specimens analyzed 10 to 20 times within a short time. It may also be estimated from the standard deviation calculated from duplicate analyses of several patient specimens within an analytical run, using Equation 2-4. Additional types of error will be introduced into the analytical process if the patient or control specimens are analyzed over a period requiring another set of calibrators or greater than one half day. For this reason, s_w is an optimistic measure of the dispersion of the analytical results.

Stability is being designed into today's instruments and methods; some instruments require infrequent calibration, eg, at 30 or 90 day intervals. The traditional definition of a run (calibrators, controls, and patient specimens) is not strictly applicable, and the meaning of s_w can be ambiguous. The National Committee for Clinical Laboratory Standards (NCCLS) has defined an analytical run as, ". . . a period of time or series of measurements, within which the accuracy and precision of the measuring system is expected to be stable . . . The length of an analytical run must be defined appropriately for the specific analytical system and specific laboratory application."[7] Nonetheless, s_w is generally still understood to reflect random variation occurring over a short time, generally less than one-half day. Our definition of an analytical run is a *group of patient specimens and the control specimens which are used to determine whether the test results on that group of patient specimens may be reported.* This definition is more practical than the NCCLS definition and is readily applied to batch testing applications.

Long-Term Variation

Increasing the period over which reference samples are analyzed increases the variation of the analytical results because other sources of variation gain importance. Brauer and Rand classified these variations as occurring from run to run, from day to day and from week to week.[5] Increased variation over time is generally related to reagent, calibrator, and operator variation; specific causes are listed in Table 2-1.

The additional variation that occurs over periods longer than one half day (the time for the generation of a run) may also be expressed as a standard deviation, which is abbreviated as s_b, or the between run component of variation. This component, s_b, may be subdivided into variation occurring *between runs*, s_{br}, and variation occurring *between days*, s_{bd}.

The components of variation can be added together as variances to yield total variance, as shown in Eqs. 2-7 and 2-8:

$$s_t^2 = s_w^2 + s_b^2, \qquad \text{Eq. 2-7}$$

and

$$s_t^2 = s_w^2 + s_{br}^2 + s_{bd}^2, \qquad \text{Eq. 2-8}$$

where
s_t = total standard deviation,
s_w = within run standard deviation,
s_b = combined between run standard deviation,

s_{br} = between run standard deviation,
s_{bd} = between day standard deviation.

The components of variation of an analytical method are estimated by performance of an analysis of variance (ANOVA) experiment,[8] a standard protocol which has been developed by the NCCLS.[9] A stable material is analyzed twice per run, in 2 runs per day for 20 days. All of the terms in Equation 2–8 are calculated. The total standard deviation estimated in this ANOVA experiment is approximately equal to the standard deviation of control results obtained by the analysis of a stable material once daily for several months (see Chapter 8). It has been estimated that 40% of the total variance (s_t^2) is observed in 1 run, 62% by 1 month, and 97% by 6 months;[10] these percentages depend on the relationships of the components in Equation 2–8.

SIGNIFICANCE TESTING

Serial control data often demonstrate trends. For example, control data frequently exhibit small month-to-month changes in their means and standard deviations. These changes can usually be explained by the uncertainty of the calculated means and standard deviations, but occasionally these changes appear excessive and can indicate that a real change has occurred in the operating characteristics of the analytical method. The magnitude of these changes can be evaluated by *significance testing.*

The significance test for the difference between two means is the *t-test*, which tests the ratio of the difference of the means to the combined standard error of the means. The t-value is calculated according to Equation 2–9:

$$t = \frac{\bar{x}_1 - \bar{x}_2}{\sqrt{\dfrac{s_1^2}{N_1^2} + \dfrac{s_2^2}{N_2^2}}}, \qquad \text{Eq. 2–9}$$

where subscripts 1 and 2 represent the 2 data sets being compared. The calculated t-value is compared to the critical t-value from Table 2–2 for the desired probability level and ($N_1 + N_2 - 2$) degrees of freedom (if s_1 is approximately equal to s_2). If the absolute value of the calculated t exceeds the critical t-value, then the difference between the means is not due to random variation alone, and is *statistically significant.*

In a typical situation, when the control data for 2 months from the

Table 2–2   Critical values of t for selected probabilities and degrees of freedom.

Degrees of freedom	p = 0.05	p = 0.01
1	12.70	63.70
2	4.30	9.92
3	3.18	5.84
4	2.78	4.60
5	2.57	4.03
6	2.45	3.71
7	2.36	3.50
8	2.31	3.36
9	2.26	3.25
10	2.23	3.17
12	2.18	3.05
14	2.14	2.98
16	2.12	2.92
18	2.10	2.88
20	2.09	2.85
30	2.04	2.75
40	2.02	2.70
60	2.00	2.66
120	1.98	2.62
∞	1.96	2.58

Abbreviations: p = probability.

Modified with permission. From Pearson ES, Hartley HO, eds. Biometrika tables for statisticians. Vol. 1, 3rd ed. Biometrika, London, Table 12.

normal level control material for a glucose method were examined, the following statistics were calculated: for March, $\bar{x}$ = 134 mg/dL, s = 2.4 mg/dL, and N = 30. For April, $\bar{x}$ = 131 mg/dL, s = 2.5 mg/ dL, and N = 29. The calculated t-value is 3.13 with 57 degrees of freedom. From Table 2–2, the critical t-value for p = 0.01 and 57 degrees of freedom is approximately 2.66. Thus, the difference between the means for March and April has less than a 1% probability of occurring due to chance alone, and the difference is statistically significant ($p < 0.01$). If the calculated t-value had been 2.32, exceeding the critical t-value for p = 0.05, but less than the critical t-value for p = 0.01, the difference between the means for March and April has less than a 5% probability of occurring due to chance alone, but more than a 1% probability of occurring due to chance alone, and the difference is statistically less significant ($p < 0.05$). If the calculated t-value in this example were 1.75, the observed difference between the means would have more than a 5% probability of occurring due to chance alone. The decision to use p = 0.01 or 0.05 for critical values depends on

21

the information being sought from the t-test, and is somewhat arbitrary.

The significance test for determining whether 2 standard deviations are significantly different is the F-test, which tests the ratio of the variance from the larger standard deviation to the variance from the smaller standard deviation against a critical F-value. The F-value is calculated according to Equation 2–10:

$$F = \frac{s_1^2}{s_2^2},$$
Eq. 2–10

where the subscripts 1 and 2 refer to the larger and smaller observed standard deviations, respectively. The calculated F-value is compared to the critical F-value in Table 2–3 according to the number of degrees of freedom for the numerator $(N_1 - 1)$ and denominator $(N_2 - 1)$. In the example using control data from March and April, if the standard deviation for March is 2.4 mg/dL, with $N = 31$, and the standard deviation for April is 3.7 mg/dL, with $N = 30$, the calculated F-value is 2.38. From Table 2–3, the critical F-value for 29 degrees of freedom for the numerator and 30 degrees of freedom for the denominator is approximately 1.84. Since the calculated F-value exceeds the critical F-value for $p = 0.05$, there is less than a 5% probability that such a large difference in standard deviations would occur due to chance alone, and the difference is statistically significant. The standard deviations for March and April really are different. If the calculated F-value had not exceeded the critical F-value, there would be more than a 5% probability that the observed difference in standard deviations could occur due to chance alone.

INHERENT BIOLOGICAL VARIATION

Cotlove,[11] Young,[12] Winkel and Statland[13] and others have measured the temporal variation of various analytes in individual normal healthy subjects (the intraindividual variation) as well as the variation of different analytes in groups of healthy subjects (the interindividual variation). For example, Cotlove, Harris, and Williams measured 15 serum constituents of 68 healthy subjects weekly for 10 to 12 weeks.[11] As in the case of the control data, an ANOVA calculation was used to derive the within individual (intraindividual) and between individual (interindividual) variation. Their estimates of the components of biologic variation, expressed in standard deviations, are shown in Table 2–4 and are compared to the standard deviation of each of the analytical methods.

Table 2–3   Critical values of F for p = 0.05 and selected degrees of freedom.

Degrees of freedom for denominator	Degrees of freedom for numerator						
	5	10	15	20	30	60	inf
5	5.05	4.74	4.62	4.56	4.50	4.43	4.36
10	3.33	2.98	2.85	2.77	2.70	2.62	2.54
15	2.90	2.54	2.40	2.33	2.25	2.16	2.07
20	2.70	2.35	2.20	2.12	2.04	1.95	1.84
30	2.53	2.16	2.01	1.93	1.84	1.74	1.62
60	2.37	1.99	1.84	1.75	1.65	1.53	1.39
∞	2.21	1.83	1.67	1.57	1.46	1.32	1.00

Abbreviations: p = probability.

Modified with permission. Biometrika tables for statisticians. Vol. 1, 3rd ed. Biometrika, London, Table 12.

For some analytes, eg, cholesterol and the enzyme aspartate aminotransferase (AST), the interindividual variances are much greater than the intraindividual variances. For other analytes, eg, electrolytes, the intraindividual and interindividual variances are approximately equal. Of more significance from the point of view of statistical quality control is that for some analytes, the inherent random variation of the analytical method is of the same magnitude as the physiologic variation. The methods used for measurement of these analytes must be monitored very carefully because increased analytic variation can give the appearance of a medically significant abnormality when none is present. Analytical performance requirements will be considered in Chapter 5.

ANALYTIC ERRORS: RANDOM AND SYSTEMATIC ERRORS

Random error is present in all observations and results in the dispersion of observations around their mean. Terms used to refer to random error are *precision, imprecision, repeatability*, and *reproducibility*. The inherent random variation of a method is termed an error because it results in disagreement between single measurements and the mean analyte concentration obtained by measuring a specimen many times. Increased random error results in increased dispersion of control specimen measurements. Any increase in random error beyond the inherent random error effectively increases the standard deviation of the method. In Figure 2–3 a frequency histogram of control measurements obtained with the inherent random error alone (without

23

Table 2–4 Comparison of the standard deviation of various analytical methods (s_a) to the intraindividual variation (s_{intra}) and the interindividual variation (s_{inter}).

Analyte	S_a	S_{intra}	S_{inter}
Sodium, mmol/L	1.7	0.0	1.12
Potassium, mmol/L	0.09	0.208	0.178
Chloride, mmol/L	1.2	1.44	1.21
CO_2, mmol/L	0.9	1.14	1.20
Calcium, mmol/L	0.085	0.043	0.071
Magnesium, mmol/L	0.04	0.013	0.052
Phosphate, mg/dL	0.22	0.259	0.380
Total protein, g/dL	0.24	0.196	0.395
Albumin, g/dL	0.18	0.160	0.264
Glucose, mg/dL	3.5	5.25	7.38
Uric acid, mg/dL	0.22	0.463	1.04
Urea nitrogen, mg/dL	1.2	1.60	2.48
Cholesterol, mg/dL	10.0	13.10	31.98
Aspartate aminotransferase, Karmen units	2.7	1.47	3.55

Abbreviations: s_a = standard deviation of analytical method, s_{intra} = intraindividual variation, s_{inter} = interindividual variation.

Modified with permission. From Cotlove E, Harris EK, Williams GZ: Biological and analytic components of variation in longterm studies of serum constituents in normal subjects. III. Physiological and medical implications. Clin Chem 16:1028-1032, 1970.

added error) is contrasted to the frequency histogram of control measurements obtained in the presence of increased random error. Causes of increased random error include instrument instability, deterioration of reagents or erroneous preparation of reagents, pipetting error, and operator error.

Systematic error refers to a tendency of the individual analytical measurements to be shifted in 1 direction from their error-free values, either higher or lower. Mathematically, the size of a systematic error can be determined from the difference between the observed mean of a set of measurements and the true mean determined when no shift is present. Figure 2–3 illustrates how control specimens demonstrate systematic error as a shift from the previous mean. When results are shifted by a constant amount regardless of the true analyte concentration, the systematic error is termed *constant error*. Constant error may be caused by a blanking error, or a chemical or spectral interference. When errors between the measured and true concentrations are

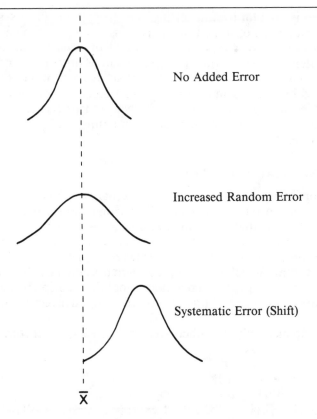

No Added Error

Increased Random Error

Systematic Error (Shift)

$\overline{X}$

Figure 2–3 Frequency histograms of control data illustrating no added error, increased random error, and systematic error.

proportional to analyte concentration, the systematic error is termed *proportional error*. A frequent cause of proportional error is miscalibration; another is side reaction of an analyte.

Analytic methods have inherent systematic error as well as inherent random error. The inherent random error is visible when reference sample statistical quality control is practiced; the inherent systematic error is not observed unless the results of reference sample testing are compared to those obtained by a method known to be free of systematic error. Thus it is possible to have good statistical quality control of a method whose inherent systematic error is unacceptably large. Before a method is used for routine testing, the acceptability of its systematic error must be demonstrated by the process of method evaluation.[14-17]

Increases in error may be intermittent or persistent in nature.[18] Intermittent errors in 1 run are independent of other runs and do not persist from 1 run to another. For example, an intermittent error may be caused by a power line surge or a bad pipet. Persistent errors are not independent from 1 run to the next, and persist until they are detected. Use of bad reagents for several runs is a typical cause of persistent error.

EXPONENTIAL SMOOTHING

Exponential smoothing offers an alternative method for deriving measures of central tendency and dispersion (mean and standard deviation). Exponential smoothing is analogous to the use of moving averages in which the oldest observation is excluded from averaging and the latest is incorporated into the average. In exponential smoothing, a new "smoothed" mean and standard deviation can be calculated for each new test result. Exponential smoothing gained recognition in laboratory quality control through its use for trend detection in control data.[19]

The exponentially smoothed average, E_t, of a series of control measurements $x_0, x_1, x_2 \ldots x_t$ is

$$
\begin{aligned}
E_t &= \alpha x_t + (1 - \alpha)E_{t-1}, \qquad\qquad \text{Eq. 2-11}\\
&= \alpha x_t + (1 - \alpha)[\alpha x_{t-1} + (1 - \alpha)E_{t-2}],\\
&= \alpha x_t + \alpha(1 - \alpha)x_{t-1} + (1 - \alpha)^2[\alpha x_{t-2} + (1 - \alpha)E_{t-3}],\\
&= \alpha x_t + \alpha(1 - \alpha)x_{t-1} + \alpha(1 - \alpha)^2 x_{t-2} + \ldots + \alpha(1 - \alpha)^2 x_{t-n}\\
&\quad + (1 - \alpha)^t x_0,\\
&= \alpha\Sigma_{n=0}^{t-1} (1 - \alpha)^n x_{t-n} + (1 - \alpha)^t x_0.
\end{aligned}
$$

The smoothed average is equal to α times the latest measurement plus $(1 - \alpha)$ times the previous average (Eq. 2-11); thus exponential smoothing is computationally very easy. The term α is called the *smoothing constant* and influences the number of observations that are effectively averaged. Expansion of Eq. 2-11 shows that the last observation is weighted by α, the second last observation is weighted by $\alpha(1 - \alpha)$, the third last by $\alpha(1 - \alpha)^2$, the fourth last by $\alpha(1 - \alpha)^3$, and so on. The smoothing constant α can have values between 0 and 1. If the value of α is 0.2 then the last observation has a weight of 0.2; the preceding observations in order of increasing age have weights of 0.16, 0.128, 0.1024, etc. Very old observations are thus weighted by very small coefficients and do not contribute significantly to the smoothed average. Newer observations, on the other hand, are weighted

Table 2–5 Smoothing constants and effective number of observations averaged (N) for exponential smoothing.

Smoothing Constant (α)	N
0.005	399
0.010	199
0.020	99
0.050	39
0.100	19
0.200	9
0.333	5
0.400	4
0.500	3
0.667	2
1.000	1

by far larger coefficients. The value of the smoothing constant α thus determines the number of observations which effectively are averaged by exponential smoothing. The relationship between α and the number of observations which are averaged, N, is shown in Equation 2–12:

$$\alpha = 2 /(N + 1). \qquad \text{Eq. 2–12}$$

Table 2–5 presents values of α and the corresponding number of observations which are effectively averaged. With a small smoothing constant, such as 0.005, the estimate behaves like the average of much past data. If the smoothing constant is large, the estimate responds rapidly to changes in pattern. Commonly used values of α of 0.1 and 0.2 correspond to the averaging of 19 and 9 control observations, respectively.

Brown[20] has described the attributes of exponential smoothing. The expected value of the exponentially smoothed observations is equal to the expected value of the observations; in other words, the current exponentially smoothed mean can be considered an average of the previous observations. The variance of the exponential average has a simple relationship to the variance of the input observations: for observations with variance s^2, the variance of the exponential average is $[\alpha/(2 - \alpha)]s^2$. Exponential smoothing is accurate. Computations are simple, and only 1 number, E_{t-1}, must be stored to calculate a new average. Exponential smoothing is flexible. No reprogramming is necessary to adjust the rate of response; only the smoothing constant need be changed.

Exponential smoothing can also be used to derive the standard deviation of the observations. This derivation uses the absolute difference of the exponentially smoothed average E_t and the next observation, x_{t+1}. If a process is in control, the differences of the exponentially smoothed average and the new observations should be 0. Both systematic error and increased random error result in increased absolute differences between the average and the new observations. The absolute differences can themselves be exponentially smoothed to derive the mean absolute difference (MAD):

$$MAD_t = \alpha|x_{t+1} - E_t| + (1 - \alpha)MAD_{t-1} . \qquad \text{Eq. 2-13}$$

The smoothed standard deviation can be calculated from the MAD:

$$s = (\pi/2)^{1/2} [(2 - \alpha)/2]^{1/2}MAD. \qquad \text{Eq. 2-14}$$

Example applications of exponential smoothing for quality control are developed in Chapters 3 and 7.

REFERENCES

1. Daniel WW: Biostatistics: a foundation for analysis in the health sciences, ed 2. John Wiley & Sons, New York, 1978.

2. Box GEP, Hunter WG, Hunter JS: Statistics for experimenters. John Wiley & Sons, New York, 1978.

3. Miller JC, Miller JN: Statistics for analytical chemistry. Ellis Horwood, Limited, Chichester, West Sussex, England, 1984.

4. Taylor JK: Quality Assurance of chemical measurements. Lewis Publishers, Chelsea, Michigan, 1987.

5. Brauer GA, Rand RN: Techniques for defining and measuring quality in clinical chemistry. In Rand RN, Eilers RJ, Lawson NS, Broughton A, eds: Quality assurance in health care: a critical appraisal of clinical chemistry. American Association for Clinical Chemistry, Washington, DC, 1980, p 207-222.

6. Buttner J, Borth R, Boutwell JH, Broughton PMG: International Federation of Clinical Chemistry provisional recommendation on quality control in clinical chemistry. I. General principles and terminology. Clin Chem 22:532-540, 1976.

7. National Committee for Clinical Laboratory Standards: Document C24-T, Internal quality control testing; principles and definitions; tentative guidelines. Villanova, Pennsylvania, 1985.

8. Bauer S, Kennedy JW: Applied statistics for the clinical laboratory: IV. Total imprecision. J Clin Lab Autom 2:129-133, 1982.

9. National Committee for Clinical Laboratory Standards: NCCLS tentative

standard EP5-T, tentative guidelines for user evaluation of precision performance of clinical chemistry devices, Subcommittee for User Evaluation of Precision of the Evaluation Protocols Area Committee, Villanova, Pa. 1983.

10. Ross JW: Evaluation of precision. In Werner M, ed: CRC handbook of clinical chemistry, vol 1. CRC Press, Boca Raton, Florida, 1982, pp 391-422.

11. Cotlove E, Harris EK, Williams GZ: Biological and analytic components of variation in long-term studies of serum constituents in normal subjects. III. Physiological and medical implications. Clin Chem 16:1028-1032, 1970.

12. Young DS, Harris EK, Cotlove E: Biological and analytic components of variation in long-term studies of serum constituents in normal subjects. IV. Results of a study designed to eliminate long-term analytic deviations. Clin Chem 17:403-410, 1971.

13. Winkel P, Statland BE: Using the subject as his own referent in assessing day-to-day changes of laboratory test results. In Hercules DM, Hieftje GM, Snyder LR, Evenson MA, eds: Contemporary topics in analytical and clinical chemistry, vol 1, Plenum Press, 1977, pp 287-317.

14. Carey RN, Garber CC: Evaluation of methods. In Kaplan LA, Pesce AJ, eds: Clinical chemistry, theory, analysis, and correlation. CV Mosby, St. Louis, 1984, pp 338-359.

15. Westgard JO: Precision and accuracy: concepts and assessment by method evaluation testing. CRC Crit Rev Clin Lab Sci, CRC Press, Boca Raton, Florida, 1981, pp 283-330.

16. Westgard JO, Carey RN, Wold S: Criteria for judging precision and accuracy in development and evaluation. Clin Chem 20:825-833, 1974.

17. Westgard JO, de Vos DJ, Hunt MR, et al: Concepts and practices in the selection and evaluation of methods, Am J Med Technol; Part I. Background and approach, 44:290-300, 1978; Part II. Experimental procedures, 44:420-430, 1978; Part III. Statistics, 44:552-571, 1978; Part IV. Decisions on acceptability, 44:727-742, 1978; Part V. Applications, 44:803-813, 1978.

18. Westgard JO, Petersen PH, Groth T: The quality-costs of an analytical process: 1. development of quality-costs models based on predictive value theory. In de Verdier CH, Aronsson T, and Nyberg A, eds: Quality control in clinical chemistry—efforts to find an efficient strategy. Scand J Clin Lab Invest 44, suppl. 172:221-227, 1984.

19. Cembrowski GS, Westgard JO, Eggert AA, Toren EC: Trend detection in control data: optimization and interpretation of Trigg's technique for trend analysis. Clin Chem 21:1396-1405, 1975.

20. Brown RG: Smoothing, forecasting and prediction of discrete time series. Prentice-Hall, Englewood-Cliffs, New Jersey, 1962.

CHAPTER THREE

Quality Control Rules

CONTROL RULES

In Chapter 1 precision and accuracy were recognized as the quality characteristics which are controlled during the routine operation of an instrument or method. Using Juran's schema for quality control (see Chapter 1), the measurement unit in the quality control process is the analytical run, which includes 1 or more control samples plus patient specimens to be reported. A control rule is used to judge whether the control results represent acceptable accuracy and precision. The control rule tests the control results against statistically defined control limits. These control limits are derived from the mean and standard deviation of control results obtained during the stable operation of an analytical method (baseline population). The control limits represent a "cutoff" beyond which results from the baseline population are expected to occur infrequently. An error condition should be suspected whenever control results are beyond their control limits.

A variety of control rules have been used to monitor the quality of laboratory analyses. One of the simplest and most popular control rules uses the mean $\pm$ 2s control limits. Only 4.5% of control results should be found outside the $\pm$ 2s limits. The lower control limit is calculated from the formula $\bar{x} - 2s$ and the upper limit from $\bar{x} + 2s$, where $\bar{x}$ and s are the long-term mean and standard deviation, respectively. Whenever a new control observation is obtained, it is compared to the mean $\pm$ 2s control limits. If an observation is outside these limits it may indicate an accuracy or precision problem.

The testing of control results against statistical control limits can be accomplished in 2 ways. The first approach requires the comparison of control observations against posted numerical control limits. The second uses a graphical approach in which control limit lines are plot-

Potassium
Level I

Date	Range 3.5 - 4.1		Action	Signature
Jan. 3	3.7			LC
Jan. 4	3.9			LC
Jan. 5	3.9			LC
Jan. 6	3.8			LC
Jan. 7	3.5			GA
Jan. 8	③.4	3.5	Repeated	GA
Jan. 9	3.6			GA
Jan. 10	3.5			LC
Jan. 11	③.3	3.4	Shift Detected	LC

Potassium
Level I

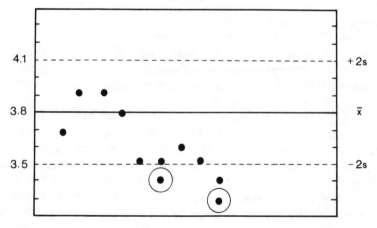

Figure 3–1 Record of daily potassium control data and its control chart representation.

ted on graph paper. Each new control observation is plotted on the graph paper; an error condition is suggested by the occurrence of a control result beyond the control limits. Figure 3–1 shows an excerpt from the record of daily potassium control data for the low-level control assayed in a physician office laboratory. The posted limits (mean ± 2s) are 3.5 to 4.1 mmol/L. There is a slow decrease in the control data which is not immediately apparent with the tabular approach. The control chart of the potassium data, also shown in Figure 3–1, shows the trend in the potassium control values. The control chart approach, while requiring the extra step of plotting the control data, allows the visualization of trends, as demonstrated in Figure 3–1. Plotting of control results can be laborious if several control levels are analyzed more often than once a shift.

There is another approach, which is a combination of the tabular and graphical approach, that we call the *tabular control chart*. A tabular control chart using the potassium control data is shown in Figure 3–2. In the usual application of the tabular control chart, control data are classified into 9 distinct categories according to their distance from the mean ($\bar{x}$): beyond $\bar{x} - 3s$, between $\bar{x} - 3s$ and $\bar{x} - 2s$, between $\bar{x} - 2s$ and $\bar{x} - 1s$, between $\bar{x} - 1s$ and $\bar{x}$, $\bar{x}$, between $\bar{x}$ and $\bar{x} + 1s$, between $\bar{x} + 1s$ and $\bar{x} + 2s$, between $\bar{x} + 2s$ and $\bar{x} + 3s$, and beyond $\bar{x} + 3s$. The tabular control chart permits recording of the control results as numbers in a manner which facilitates the detection of trends. The use of the tabular control chart for isoenzyme analyses has been described by Broome et al.[1]

Some control rules incorporate multiple control or patient observations. Some require numerical manipulation of the observations before being compared to statistical limits. Descriptions of many of the popular control rules are presented in this chapter along with their advantages and limitations.[2,3]

Because of the large number of control rules and their diverse implementations, Westgard devised a shorthand notation for representing these rules.[2] The notation for the control rules is in the form A_L, where A is the abbreviation for a particular statistic or the number of control observations, and L is the control limit. The abbreviation 1_{2s} refers to the control rule which uses mean ± 2s limits. Short descriptions of the more commonly used control rules are presented in Table 3–1.

PERFORMANCE CHARACTERISTICS OF CONTROL RULES

Computer Simulation Studies: Probabilities for False Rejection and Error Detection

The error detection capabilities of control rules have been evaluated by Westgard and coworkers using computer simulation techniques.[2,4]

Level I

Date	3.25 x̄-3s	3.5 x̄-2s	3.65 x̄-1s	3.8 x̄	3.95 x̄+1s	4.1 x̄+2s	4.25 x̄+3s	Action / Signature	
Jan. 3			3.7						LC
Jan. 4					3.9				LC
Jan. 5					3.9				LC
Jan. 6				3.8					LC
Jan. 7		3.5							GA
Jan. 8	(3.4)	3.5						Repeated	GA
Jan. 9		3.6							GA
Jan. 10		3.5							LC
Jan. 11	(3.3) 3.4							Shift Detected	LC

Figure 3–2   Tabular control chart of the data of Figure 3–1.

The first step in a quality control simulation program is the calculation of control limits (for the control rule being tested) based on a selected mean and standard deviation. The program then generates a series of baseline control results with a gaussian (normal) distribution using the selected mean and standard deviation. These simulated baseline control results are tested against the calculated control limits. Results exceeding these limits are classified as "false rejections," since they are actually from the baseline population, and no error condition is present. The *probability of false rejection*, P_{fr}, is calculated by dividing the number of control results exceeding the limits by the total number of control results.

The impact of analytical error, either systematic error or random error, is demonstrated by generating a new series of control results with a different mean (systematic error or shift) or a larger standard deviation (increased random error). The new control results are tested against the *original* control limits. Control results exceeding these limits are classified as true rejections, or error detections. The *probability of error detection*, P_{ed}, is calculated by dividing the number of control results exceeding the control limits by the total number of control

33

Table 3-1 Popular control rules for the interpretation of reference sample measurements.

1_{2s}	Reject an analytical run (or warn of analytical problem) when 1 control observation exceeds the $\bar{x} \pm 2s$ control limits; usually used as a warning.
$1_{2.5s}$	Reject an analytical run when 1 control observation exceeds the $\bar{x} \pm 2.5s$ control limits.
1_{3s}	Reject an analytical run when 1 control observation exceeds the $\bar{x} \pm 3s$ control limits.
$1_{3.5s}$	Reject an analytical run when 1 control observation exceeds the $\bar{x} \pm 3.5s$ control limits.
2_{2s}	Reject an analytical run when 2 consecutive control observations are on the same side of the mean and exceed either the $\bar{x} + 2s$ or $\bar{x} - 2s$ control limits.
4_{1s}	Reject an analytical run when 4 consecutive control observations are on the same side of the mean and exceed either the $\bar{x} + 1s$ or $\bar{x} - 1s$ control limits.
10_x	Reject an analytical run when 10 consecutive control observations are on the same side of the mean.
R_{4s}	Reject an analytical run if the range or difference between the maximum and minimum control observation exceeds 4s.
$\bar{X}_{0.01}$	Reject an analytical run if the mean of the last N control observations exceeds the control limits that give a 1% frequency of false rejection ($P_{fr} = 0.01$).
$R_{0.01}$	Reject an analytical run if the range of the last N control observations exceeds the control limits that give a 1% frequency of false rejection ($P_{fr} = 0.01$).

results. Histograms expected for the baseline population and the populations after introduction of increased random and systematic errors are shown in Figure 3-3.

In order to obtain truly representative P_{ed} values, approximately 400 to 1000 analytical runs must be simulated at each error level (eg, no added error, shift = 1s, shift = 2s, shift = 3s, etc).

Power Function Graphs

Finally, the data are summarized graphically by a power function graph, on which the probability of rejection (equivalent to the proportion of rejections) is plotted against the size of error. Figure 3-4 shows computer-generated power function graphs for the 1_{2s} control rule, one for the detection of systematic error, and the other for the

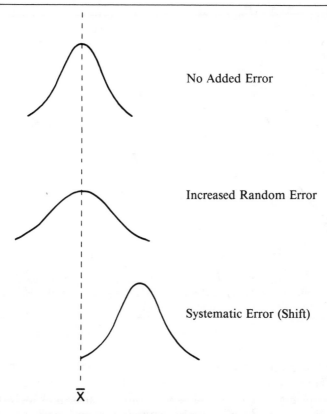

Figure 3–3 Idealized frequency histograms of control data showing no added analytical error, increased random error and systematic error.

detection of random error. The lines are not smooth due to the imprecision of the simulation process. These power function curves were obtained by simulating the analysis of single control specimens and comparing their results to the $\bar{x} \pm 2s$ control limits. The x axis ranges are different for the 2 graphs. The systematic error power function graph begins at 0s (no shift; only inherent random error present) and extends to 5s (corresponding to a shift of 5s). For the random error power function graph, the x axis begins at 1s (standard deviation = 1 times baseline standard deviation; only inherent random error present) and extends to 5s (corresponding to an increase of the standard deviation to 5 times the original standard deviation).

The power function for the 1_{2s} rule in Figure 3–4 may be applied

Probability

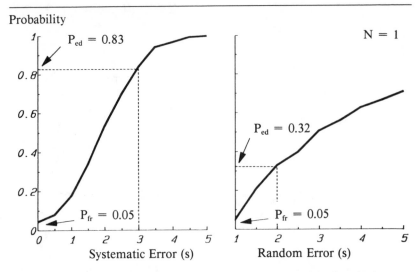

Figure 3–4 Power function graphs for the 1_{2s} control rule using single control observations for systematic and random error. Probability of rejection is plotted against the magnitude of error.

to a glucose method which produces control observations with a mean of 100 and standard deviation of 3 mg/dL. The systematic error represented in Figure 3–4 would range from 0 mg/dL (0s) to 15 mg/dL (5s). A systematic error of 3s corresponds to a shift of 9 mg/dL. The x axis for the random error power functions would range from 3 mg/dL (1s) to 15 mg/dL (5 × s). A random error of 2s corresponds to a doubling of the standard deviation to 6 mg/dL.

The probability of rejection, plotted on the y axis, ranges from 0 to 1. The probability of false rejection, P_{fr}, is derived from the y intercept. The P_{fr} can be determined from either the systematic or random error power function graph. It corresponds to the situation where there is no systematic error, and the only random error is the inherent random error of the method. The P_{fr} for the 1_{2s} control rule with 1 control observation is approximately 0.05 or 5%, which can be verified with the probability theory presented in Chapter 2. You will recall that in the absence of additional analytical error, the use of the mean ± 2s limits will result in 95.5% of the control observations being within the control limits. The probability of observing a single control observation outside these limits will thus be 100 − 95.5, or 4.5%. Of course, as more control observations are examined, there is a higher probability that at least 1 of these control observations will be outside the mean ± 2s control limits. The probability that at least 1 of N control observations will be outside the control limits can be calculated from the formula.

$$P_{fr}(\%) = 100 \times (1 - .955^N).$$ Eq. 3–1

The probability of error detection, P_{ed}, can be determined for any size error. The size of the error is first located on the x axis, and a vertical line is drawn from there to intersect the power function curve. From this intersection, a horizontal line is drawn to the y axis. The P_{ed} is the value of the probability on the y axis. Thus, in Figure 3–4, with the 1_{2s} control rule and 1 control per run, the P_{ed} for a 3s shift (9 mg/dL) is 0.83, and the P_{ed} for a random error of 2s (standard deviation = 6 mg/dL) is 0.32. The P_{ed} can be verified by probability calculations; however, these calculations become complex as several rules are applied simultaneously.

Optimal Power Function Curve

Power function curves present so much information in a single graph that it is easy to be overwhelmed. To provide a perspective for interpreting power functions, we have presented an idealized power function curve in Figure 3–5. Small-sized errors, either shifts or increased random error, are unavoidable and will occur despite rigorous preventive maintenance and troubleshooting. In general, quality control rules should not reject analytical runs with small analytical errors. For many common chemistry, hematology, and coagulation analytes measured on today's highly precise analyzers, it is not usually necessary to reject analytical runs with systematic errors of less than 1.0s or random errors less than 1.5 times the original random error. The probability of detecting these small errors for rejection purposes should be approximately 0. The probability of detecting larger errors should be close to 1.00. There are certain analytes for which it is important to detect smaller shifts and increases in random error, ie, those analytes for which the standard deviation of the analytical method is of the same magnitude as the interindividual or intraindividual standard deviation (how much error is allowable will be covered more thoroughly in Chapters 5 and 8).

As the reader studies power function curves, he or she should begin to recognize rules which are overly sensitive to small levels of analytical error. A P_{fr} greater than 5% is usually unacceptable and results in large numbers of rejected runs with no significant error. Similarly, control

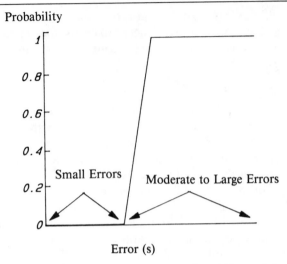

Probability

Figure 3–5 Ideal power function curve, $P_{fr} = 0$ and $P_{ed} = 0$ for small errors, $P_{ed} = 1$ for moderate to large errors.

rules yielding a P_{ed} greater than 10% to 15% for small errors should not be used for rejection purposes. Rather, they may be used to alert the analyst to a problem which may need to be corrected eventually. The reader should also begin to classify control rules into 2 categories, those which are sensitive to moderate to large systematic error, and those sensitive to moderate to large random error.

CONTROL RULES USING SINGLE OUTLYING OBSERVATIONS

The following control rules require the comparison of successive *single* control observations to control limits determined from the mean and standard deviation. The concise form of the control rule is 1_{ns} (1 refers to the number of control observations; *ns* corresponds to the control limits about the mean, with *n* referring to the number of standard deviations and *s* the standard deviation).

1_{2s} Rule

The power function curves for the 1_{2s} control rule are shown in Figure 3–6. The number of control observations within a run can be

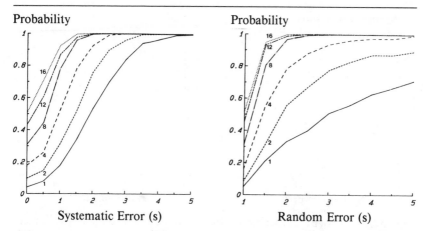

Figure 3-6 Power function graphs for the 1_{2s} control rule for systematic and random error. The numbers correspond to the number of control observations.

replicates of the same control material or the total number of results for several materials tested within the run. The P_{fr} is unacceptably high for 2 or more control observations. For example, if the 1_{2s} control rule is used with 2 control observations per analytical run, there is approximately a 10% chance that at least 1 of the 2 controls will exceed the $\bar{x} \pm 2s$ control limits *in the absence of added analytical error.* This rejection rate is much higher in the presence of small shifts and small increases in random error.

The high false alarm rate of the 1_{2s} control rule has conditioned most technologists to duly note the occurrence of the rule violation, but not follow it with any investigative or corrective action. The most impressive examples of the 1_{2s} control rule's high P_{fr} are associated with its application on multichannel chemistry and hematology analyzers. For example, a multichannel chemistry analyzer which generates 12 different results from a single control specimen will produce an outlying control result on 45% of the occasions that the control is run. Clearly, the 1_{2s} control rule is inappropriate in most situations when more than 1 control observation is used, although its popularity in clinical laboratories continues. Its use for rejection purposes should be limited to situations where a high P_{ed} is required and only 1 control can be analyzed.

As the number of controls included in each analytical run is increased, rules with wider limits must be selected in order to maintain

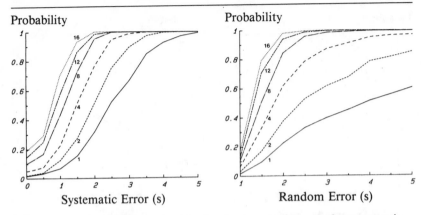

Figure 3–7 Power function graphs for the $1_{2.5s}$ control rule for systematic error and random error. The numbers correspond to the number of control observations.

an acceptable P_{fr}. As the limits are widened from $\pm$ 2s to $\pm$ 2.5s, $\pm$ 3s, and $\pm$ 3.5s, the P_{fr} and P_{ed} are both reduced.

$1_{2.5s}$ Rule

Use of the $1_{2.5s}$ control rule to control clinical chemistry determinations was originally proposed by Blum.[5] Its power function curves are shown in Figure 3–7. The P_{fr} is approximately 2% for N = 1, 4% for N = 2, and 7% for N = 4. Use of this control rule with an N of 4 or greater will result in an unacceptable false rejection rate. When 2 controls are used, the P_{ed} for a shift of 2s is reduced from 0.76 for the 1_{2s} rule to 0.50 for the $1_{2.5s}$ rule. The P_{ed} for a doubling of random error is decreased from 0.54 to 0.38.

1_{3s} Rule

The 1_{3s} control rule is probably the most popular control rule. The power function curves for this control rule are shown in Figure 3–8. The P_{fr} is very low, approximately 0.3% for 1 control observation and 5% for 16 control observations. Unfortunately, the P_{ed} is commensurately low for a small N. For example, for 2 control observations, a 2s shift is detected with a probability of 30%, and a doubling of the random error is detected with a probability of 24%. For N = 4, the

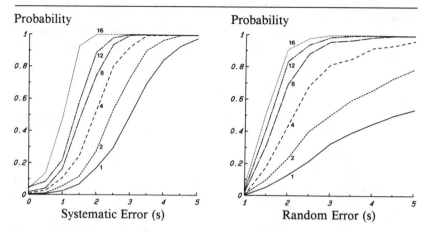

Figure 3-8 Power function graphs for the 1_{3s} control rule for systematic and random error. The numbers correspond to the number of control observations.

detection of systematic error appears optimal, but the P_{ed} remains low for the detection of large random errors.

$1_{3.5s}$ Rule

The $1_{3.5s}$ rule has even lower P_{fr} values, from 0.0003 for 1 control observation to 0.01 for 16 control observations. The P_{ed} for 2 controls for a shift of 2s and doubling of random error are 0.15 and 0.14, respectively. Power function curves are shown in Figure 3-9. Clearly, use of this rule is limited to situations in which only very large errors must be detected.

CONTROL RULES USING COUNTS OF CONSECUTIVE OBSERVATIONS (COUNTING RULES)

The "counting rules" are simple to implement because they require only the counting of consecutive control observations occurring on the same side of the mean and exceeding a specified minimum difference from the mean. The concise form of the control rule is N_{ns}, where N refers to the number of consecutive control observations, with the minimum distance being expressed as multiples of the standard deviation (ns). Because these rules require consecutive observations on

41

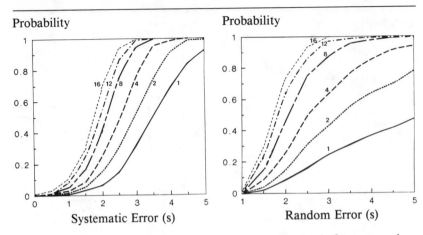

Figure 3–9 Power function graphs for the $1_{3.5s}$ control rule for systematic and random error. The numbers correspond to the number of control observations.

one side of the mean to signal a rule violation, they detect systematic error far more readily than random error.

Control rules which incorporate 2 or more observations can be applied within or across control materials. Two or more control levels are generally used for quality control, with each level considered a separate control material. If a control rule considers control observations from only 1 control material, then that control rule is used within control materials. If a control rule uses control observations from multiple control materials, then that control rule is used across control materials. Similarly, some control rules may be applied to control observations obtained within an analytical run or across analytical runs. Applying a control rule within a run means that only control observations from that run are evaluated. Applying a control rule across runs means that 1 or more control observations from the current run are evaluated along with 1 or more control observations from the previous run or runs.

2_{2s} Rule

The most commonly used counting rule is the 2_{2s}, which rejects when 2 consecutive control observations are on the same side of the mean and at least 2s away from the mean. Violations of this rule are illustrated in Figure 3–10. This rule is used by many analysts when

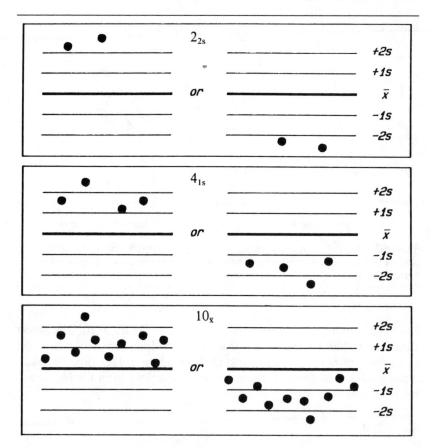

Figure 3–10   Control charts illustrating violations of the 2_{2s} control rule (top), 4_{1s} control rule (middle) and 10_x control rule (bottom).

they rerun a control which has exceeded its 2s limits. If the control result again exceeds its 2s limits, then the analytical run is usually rejected. The power functions for the 2_{2s} control rule are shown in Figure 3–11. A very low P_{fr} is shown. The P_{ed} for systematic error is optimal for N = 8 and is almost adequate for N = 4. The P_{ed} for random error is low for even large N.

4_{1s} Rule

The 4_{1s} rule rejects when 4 consecutive control observations are on the same side of the mean and at least 1s away from the mean. Vio-

43

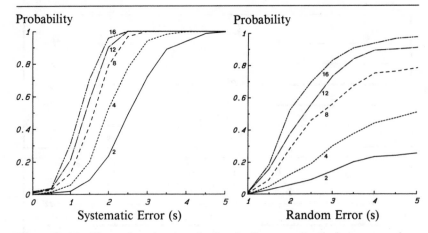

Figure 3–11 Power function graphs for the 2_{2s} control rule for systematic and random error. The numbers correspond to the number of control observations.

lations of the 4_{1s} control rule are illustrated in Figure 3–10. The power function graphs for the 4_{1s} control rule show high sensitivity to small systematic errors, especially with an N of 12 or greater (Figure 3–12). The capability to detect random error is quite low, even for 16 control observations.

$10_{\bar{x}}$ Rule

The $10_{\bar{x}}$ control rule requires 10 consecutive control observations to be on the same side of the mean. Violations of the control rule are illustrated in Figure 3–10. The power function graphs for the $10_{\bar{x}}$ control rule show very high sensitivity to small systematic errors, even with as few as 16 control observations (Figure 3–13). The ability to detect random error is almost nil. Because of the high sensitivity to small shifts, which are very common in today's analyzers, the $10_{\bar{x}}$ rule's most useful function is to indicate a need for eventual recalibration or maintenance. In most circumstances, it should not be used to reject analytical runs.

"PROPORTION" CONTROL RULES

If 2 or more control observations are evaluated together, control rules can be devised which require a specific proportion of observations

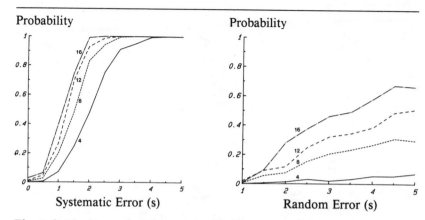

Figure 3–12 Power function graphs for the 4_{1s} control rule for systematic and random error. The numbers correspond to the number of control observations.

to exceed their control limits. For example, Westgard studied the use of 3 levels of control material for the quality control of blood gas analyzers. He proposed a rule which required 2 of the last 3 controls to exceed the $\bar{x} \pm 2s$ control limits.[6] Westgard abbreviated this control rule as the $(2 \text{ of } 3)_{2s}$ control rule. Carey has studied the use of the $(3 \text{ of } 8)_{2s}$ control rule for the retrospective quality control of an automated multichannel chemistry analyzer.[7] These "proportion" control rules simplify the evaluation of control data across controls; no computation is necessary. Both random and systematic error can be detected with these rules. Under certain conditions the power of the proportion control rule approaches that of the combination of the mean and range rules. As the number of control observations increases, so does the number of possible combinations of proportion rules. The performance characteristics of these combinations have not been well documented.

CONTROL RULES EMPLOYING STATISTICS OF CONTROL OBSERVATIONS

The next 3 control rules, the range (R), mean ($\bar{X}$), and chi-square (χ^2), require the calculation of a statistic—the range, mean, or standard deviation, respectively—before being compared to a control limit. These 3 rules can have their P_{fr} fixed at a predetermined level. The P_{fr} follows the abbreviation of the rule. Thus $R_{0.01}$ corresponds to the range rule

Probability

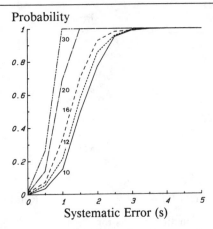

Systematic Error (s)

Figure 3–13 Power function graphs for the 10_x control rule for systematic error. The numbers correspond to the number of control observations.

whose P_{fr} is 0.01; similarly, $\bar{X}_{0.002}$ corresponds to the mean rule whose P_{fr} is 0.002. The most common implementation of the range rule, the R_{4s}, does not have a constant P_{fr}. Rather, the range of a group of control observations is calculated and then compared with the control limits, 4s. Because calculations of the mean and standard deviation are difficult by hand, the mean and chi-square rules are usually implemented with computers.

R_{4s} Rule

The R_{4s} rule requires an analytical run to be rejected when the range, or difference between the highest and lowest control observations within the run, to exceed 4s. Typical implementations of the rule require 1 control observation to exceed a limit of $\bar{x} + 2s$ and another control observation to exceed the $\bar{x} - 2s$ limit. That is, each observation is out by at least 2s, but in opposite directions, making a total difference of at least 4s. An example of a R_{4s} violation is shown in Figure 3–14. The R_{4s} rule may be defined as requiring that the range be exceeded either by 2 consecutive control results or by any 2 control results within the run (for example the 1st and 3rd of 3 control results). Power function curves for the latter definition of the R_{4s} rule are shown in Figure 3–15. The P_{fr} is acceptably low for 2 to 4 observations; however, for more than 4 observations, the P_{fr} is excessive.

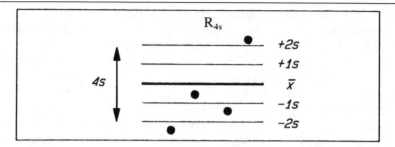

Figure 3–14   Control chart illustrating a violation of the R_{4s} control rule.

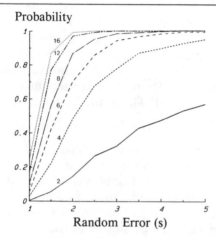

Figure 3–15   Power function graphs for the R_{4s} control rule for random error. The numbers correspond to the number of control observations.

R_{Pfr} Rule

The disadvantage of the R_{4s} rule is that when more than 4 observations are gathered, there is an unacceptably high probability that their range will exceed 4s even in the absence of increased random error. There is another set of range rules for which the range increases with an increasing N. By appropriately adjusting the acceptable range, the P_{fr} can be fixed at a predefined level. These rules are abbreviated R_{Pfr}. The $R_{0.01}$ rule corresponds to the range rule for which the probability of false rejection is set to 1.0%. For 2 observations, the acceptable range is 3.64s; for 3 observations, the range increases to 4.12s;

and for 4 observations, the acceptable range is 4.40s. Factors for calculating control limits for ranges for various N and P_{fr} are tabulated in Table 3–2. Figure 3–16 shows the performance of the $R_{0.05}$, $R_{0.01}$, and the $R_{0.002}$ rules; the P_{fr} is fixed at 5%, 1%, and 0.2%, respectively. The $R_{0.01}$ and $R_{0.002}$ rules appear to perform similarly; both control rules demonstrate low probabilities of detecting small increases in random error. The $R_{0.05}$ rule, on the other hand, will detect small increases in random error with fairly high probability. Its use should be limited to situations in which such high sensitivity to random error is required.

$\overline{X}_{Pfr}$ Rule

Just as the control limits for the range rule can be adjusted to provide a constant P_{fr}, regardless of N, the limits for the mean rule can be similarly adjusted. In Chapter 2, we showed that confidence limits for the mean could be expressed as multiples of the standard error of the mean $(s/\sqrt{N})$. As more observations are gathered (increased N), the uncertainty about the mean decreases and the acceptable limits for the mean are narrowed. The limits for the mean are expressed as

$$\text{Limits} = \overline{x} \pm \text{Multiplier} \times (s/\sqrt{N}). \qquad \text{Eq. 3–2}$$

The multiplier determines the confidence limits for the mean. The values $\overline{x}$ and s correspond to the long-term mean and standard deviation, respectively. In the usual implementation of the mean rule, the mean of every N control observation is computed and compared to the limits determined by Equation 3–2. A problem in the analytical process would be indicated by a mean outside of these limits. A multiplier of 2.58 corresponds to the 99% confidence limits for the mean. Thus, if the control limits were set to $\overline{x} \pm 2.58 \times s/\sqrt{N}$, only 1% of the means would be outside of the control limits in the absence of analytical error. Other multipliers which are commonly used for the calculation of control limits include 1.96(P_{fr} = 5%), 2.00(P_{fr} = 4.5%), 3.00(P_{fr} = 0.3%), and 3.09(P_{fr} = 0.2%).

Figure 3–17 shows power function curves for the $\overline{X}_{0.05}$, $\overline{X}_{0.01}$, $\overline{X}_{0.002}$ control rules, which have P_{fr} values of 5%, 1%, and 0.2%, respectively. As the P_{fr} decreases, the curves are shifted to the right. The power function curves of the $\overline{X}_{0.05}$ indicate a high P_{ed} for small shifts with an N of 4 or greater. The performance characteristics of the $\overline{X}_{0.01}$ and $\overline{X}_{0.002}$ rules for 2 or 4 observations resemble the optimal power function curve (Figure 3–5). However, when 12 or more observations are averaged, the probability of detecting small shifts becomes quite high.

Mean rules have other disadvantages as well. It is computationally

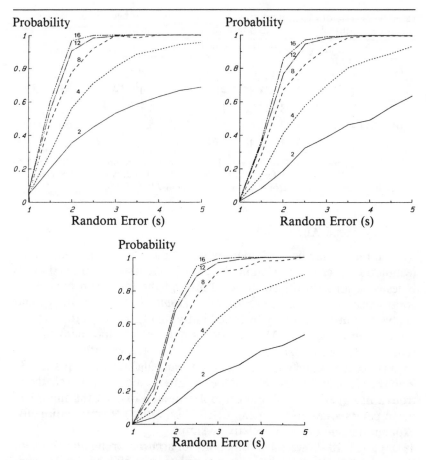

Figure 3–16 Power function graphs for the (A) $R_{0.05}$, (B) $R_{0.01}$ and (C) $R_{0.002}$ control rules for random error. The numbers correspond to the number of control observations.

cumbersome to vary the number of replicate control results included in the calculation of the mean, because the control limits vary with the number of replicates. Mean rules can only be applied across controls by computing the mean z-score, and using the above multipliers themselves for the limits for the mean z-score (see Chapter 2 for discussion of the z-score). Thus, practical use of mean rules is limited to control procedures which involve testing the same relatively large number of replicates of each control material in each run.

Table 3-2 Factors for calculating control limits for ranges from standard deviations: control limit = standard deviation × factor.

P_{fr}	Number of Control Observations									
	2	3	4	5	6	8	10	12	16	20
0.05	2.77	3.31	3.63	3.86	4.03	4.29	4.47	4.62	4.85	5.01
0.025	3.17	3.68	3.98	4.20	4.36	4.61	4.79	4.92		
0.01	3.64	4.12	4.40	4.60	4.76	4.99	5.16	5.29	5.50	5.65
0.001	4.65	5.06	5.31	5.48	5.62	5.82	5.97	6.09		

Modified with permission. From Westgard JO, Groth T, Aronsson T, Falk H, de Verdier C-H: Performance characteristics of rules for internal quality control: probabilities for false rejection and error detection. Clin Chem 23:1857–1867, 1977.

Accuracy Trend Analysis

The mean may be computed by use of the exponential smoothing techniques described in Chapter 2. The exponentially smoothed mean is tested against limits constructed around the long-term mean in a control procedure termed *accuracy trend analysis*. With accuracy trend analysis, control data may be tested individually, as they are received, rather than in batches. Most modern analyzers produce control data sequentially, rather than in batches. Limits for the smoothed mean are calculated analogously to those of the mean rule given in Equation 3–2 above.[8] The value for the number of observations, N, is calculated from α in Equation 2–10. For example, for an α of 0.10, the smoothed mean corresponds to the mean of 19 observations. Computationally, exponential smoothing is relatively simple.

Figure 3–18 shows power functions for accuracy trend analysis with the exponentially smoothed mean tested against 99% and 99.8% confidence limits. The smoothing coefficient is $\alpha = 0.1$ with the 99% control limits being $\bar{x} \pm 2.58 \times (s/\sqrt{19})$ and the 99.8% control limits being $\bar{x} \pm 3.09 \times (s/\sqrt{19})$. Figure 3–18 shows that the P_{fr} is unacceptably high when more than 20 observations are exponentially smoothed and compared to the 99% confidence limits. While use of the 99.8% limits results in an acceptably low P_{fr} even when 30 observations are averaged, shifts of small magnitude are reliably detected, some of which may not be clinically important.

Rather than comparing the exponentially smoothed mean to statistical limits, it is advantageous to compare the mean to limits which have been determined to be clinically relevant. Thus if it has been established that a shift of 1.25s can result in clinically misleading results (see Chapter 5), the error limits can be set to the mean ± 1.25s.

50

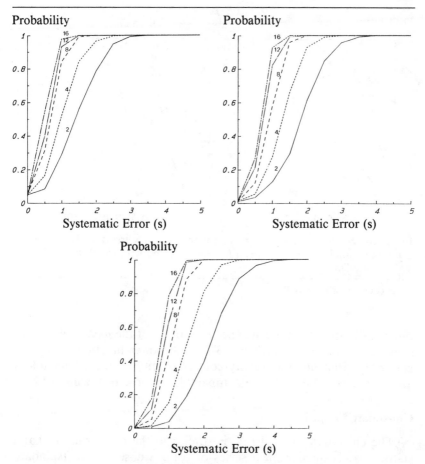

Figure 3–17   Power function graphs for the (A) $\bar{X}_{0.05}$ (B) $\bar{X}_{0.01}$ and (C) $\bar{X}_{0.002}$ control rules for systematic error. The numbers correspond to the number of control observations.

If an exponentially smoothed mean exceeds these limits, there will be a high probability that the shifted mean is clinically different from the usual mean. Figure 3–19 shows the power functions for accuracy trend analysis ($\alpha = 0.1$) with the exponentially smoothed mean tested against the mean $\pm$ 1.25s limits. As more and more observations are incorporated into the exponential smoothing, the probability of detecting a shift greater than 1.25s approaches 100%. The P_{fr} is 0 and the P_{ed} is small for a shift of less than 1.25s. The power function curves of ex-

51

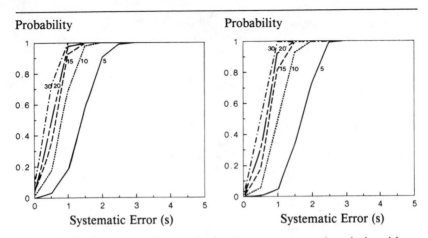

Figure 3–18 Power function graphs for the accuracy trend analysis, with the exponentially smoothed mean ($\alpha = 0.1$) tested with (A) 99% and (B) 99.8% confidence limits.

(Data courtesy of P Douville)

ponentially smoothed means approach those of the ideal power function curve illustrated in Figure 3–5. The power function curves for Bull's algorithm for the quality control of multichannel hematology analyzers (see Chapter 9) are comparable to those of Figure 3–19.

Chi-square (χ^2_{Pfr}) Rule

The chi-square control rule is similar to the mean rule in that a statistic is obtained from a series of control observations (standard deviation), and is then evaluated with a statistical test to determine whether it is statistically different from the established statistic. The statistical test employed is the chi-square test. The formula for the chi-square value is

$$\chi^2 = \frac{s_{wr}^2(N-1)}{s_{lt}^2},$$

Eq. 3–3

where

s_{wr} = standard deviation of the control observations within the analytical run which is being tested,

s_{lt} = typical within-run standard deviation.

The χ^2 value is then compared to the critical chi-square value for the appropriate N and confidence level.[9]

Probability

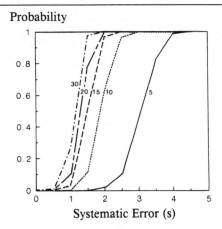

Systematic Error (s)

Figure 3-19 Power function graphs for the accuracy trend analysis with the exponentially smoothed mean ($\alpha = 0.1$) tested against the $\bar{x} \pm 1.25s$ control limits.

(Data courtesy of P Douville)

When the limits for χ^2 rules and range rules are calculated for an equivalent P_{fr}, their power functions are almost superimposable. Power function graphs for $\chi^2_{0.05}$, $\chi^2_{0.01}$, and $\chi^2_{0.005}$ rules are shown in Figure 3-20. Just as for the $\bar{X}_{0.05}$ rule, the power function curves of the $\chi^2_{0.05}$ indicate a high P_{ed} for small increases in random error with an N of 4 or greater. Similarly, the probability of detecting small increases in random error is very high with 8 or more observations when the $\chi^2_{0.01}$ and $\chi^2_{0.005}$ control rules are applied. For 2 and 4 control observations, there appears very little difference between the performance of the $\chi^2_{0.01}$ and $\chi^2_{0.005}$ control rules.

Precision Trend Analysis

As in the case of the mean, the standard deviation may be computed with exponential smoothing techniques (Chapter 2). The χ^2 test can then be used to evaluate whether the exponentially smoothed standard deviation is significantly different from the usual standard deviation. The performance characteristics of the control rule using the χ^2 test to evaluate the exponentially smoothed standard deviation are shown in Figure 3-21. The left graph shows power function curves for precision trend analysis using the 99% confidence limits. The P_{fr} levels are high and are comparable to the P_{fr} of the accuracy trend analysis

53

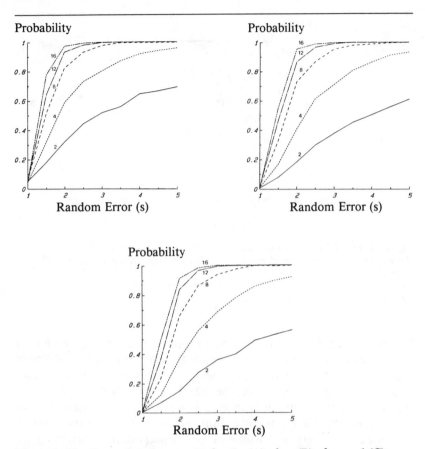

Figure 3–20 Power function graphs for the (A) $\chi^2_{0.05}$ (B) $\chi^2_{0.01}$ and (C) $\chi^2_{0.005}$ control rules for random error. The numbers correspond to the number of control observations.

of Figure 3–18. Because of the high probability of detecting small random error when statistically derived limits are used, it is preferable to compare the exponentially smoothed standard deviation to the clinically relevant standard deviation. Figure 3–21 shows power function curves for precision trend analysis with the exponentially smoothed standard deviation being compared to twice the usual standard deviation (right graph). If more than 15 specimens are averaged, there is greater than a 50% probability of detecting a random error of 2s. The P_{fr}, however, is 0 and the probability of detecting small increases in random error is low.

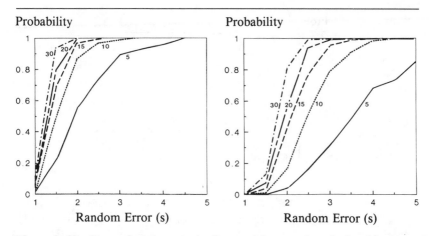

Figure 3–21 Power function graphs for precision trend analysis with the exponentially smoothed standard deviation ($\alpha = 0.01$) tested against the 99% limits (left) and 2s (right).

(Data courtesy of P Douville)

Cusum (Cumulative Summation) Rule

In cumulative summation, differences between the long-term mean and consecutive control observations are calculated and summed. In the absence of systematic error, the differences between the mean and the control observations should be randomly distributed about 0 with their sum (the cumulative sum) being close to 0. In the presence of systematic error, the differences between the mean and the control observations are consistently higher or lower than 0. The result is a cumulative sum which grows in magnitude, with the sign of the sum reflecting the direction of the systematic error. In the traditional implementation of cusum, the cumulative sums are plotted against time. A plastic or paper template called a V mask is placed over the cusum plot and is used to assess the angle and thus the magnitude (and statistical significance) of any progressively increasing or decreasing sum. The use of cumulative summation in the clinical laboratory has been minimal, being largely limited to hematology applications,[10] probably because of the requirement for calculating and plotting the cusums and the somewhat subjective interpretation of the cumulative summation trends using the V mask.

There is another approach to detecting significant trends in cumulative sums, the decision limit cusum[11] which was described by

55

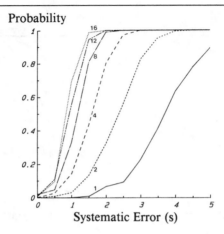

Figure 3-22   Power function graphs for the CS$^{1.0s}_{2.7s}$ control rules for systematic error. The numbers correspond to the number of control observations.

Westgard et al in 1977. Westgard's approach requires 2 different sets of control limits for the long-term mean, an inner set to evaluate individual observations and commence the cumulative summation process, and an outer set to evaluate the cumulative sum. The decision limit control rule is abbreviated CS^i_o where the superscript i stands for the inner limit and the subscript o stands for the outer limit.

Decision limit cusum works in the following manner: First, all control observations are compared, 1 at a time, to the inner control limits. If the control observations are within the inner limits, nothing is done. If a control observation occurs outside an inner limit, cumulative summation of the differences is started. The differences of individual observations are calculated by subtracting the inner control limit first exceeded in this series from the individual control observation. The differences are summed until they exceed the outer control limit (indicating an error) or until the cumulative sum changes sign, which indicates the end of the cumulative summation process.

Figure 3-22 shows a family of power function curves for the CS$^{1.0s}_{2.7s}$ control rule. Cumulative summation is started only if a control observation exceeds 1.0s. An error is indicated if the sum of the differences between the individual control observations and the inner limits exceeds the outer control limits 2.7s. The power functions indicate significant probability of detecting shifts of 0.5s when 12 or more ob-

56

servations are used. Otherwise, the performance characteristics are excellent.

Many different quality control rules may be used to analyze control data. The power function curves provide an approach to evaluating their efficacy. Control rules with high P_{fr} should not be used. Thus, the 1_{2s} control rule should not be used with 2 or more observations. Rules with a high P_{ed} for small errors either should not be used or should be used only to indicate that eventual correction may be necessary. Many of the control rules can only detect the presence of 1 type of error, eg, the counting rules for systematic error, R_{4s} for random error. Thus for the efficient detection of errors, rules should be combined, with at least 1 rule sensitive to random error and another sensitive to systematic error. In the next chapter, combinations of control rules will be described.

REFERENCES

1. Broome HE, Cembrowski GS, Kahn SN, Martin PL, Patrick CA: Implementation and use of a manual multi-rule quality control procedure. Lab Med 16:533-537, 1985.

2. Westgard JO, Groth T, Aronsson T, Falk H, de Verdier C-H: Performance characteristics of rules for internal quality control: probabilities for false rejection and error detection. Clin Chem 23:1857-1867, 1977.

3. Westgard JO, Groth T: Power functions for statistical control rules. Clin Chem 25:394-400, 1979.

4. Groth T, Falk H, Westgard JO: An interactive computer simulation program for the design of statistical control procedures in clinical chemistry. Comput Programs Biomed 13:73-86, 1981.

5. Blum AS: Computer evaluation of statistical procedures, and a new quality-control statistical procedure. Clin Chem 31:206-212, 1985.

6. Westgard JO, Groth T: Assessment of the performance characteristics of a blood gas quality control program by use of an interactive computer simulation program. Clin Chem 26:699, 1980.

7. Carey RN, Beebe S, Barry PL, Westgard JO: Assessment of performance characteristics of some quality control rules for retrospective analysis of control data from the IL 508 chemistry analyzer. Clin Chem 31:1017, 1985.

8. Westgard JO, Groth T: Design and evaluation of statistical control procedures: applications of a computer "quality control simulator" program. Clin Chem 17:1536-1545, 1981.

9. Table C, Percentage points of the χ^2 distribution. In Duncan AJ: Quality control and industrial statistics, ed 4. Richard D. Irwin, Homewood, Illinois, 1974.

10. Cavill I, Ricketts C, Fisher J, Walpole B: An evaluation of two methods of laboratory quality control. Am J Clin Pathol 72:624-627, 1979.
11. Westgard JO, Groth T, Aronsson T, de Verdier C-H: A combined Shewhart-cusum control chart for improved quality control in clinical chemistry. Clin Chem 23:1881-1887, 1977.

CHAPTER FOUR

Quality Control Procedures

RATIONALE FOR COMBINING RULES

Most quality control rules tend to detect either random or systematic error; few control rules have adequate sensitivity for the detection of both types of error. Moreover, when fewer than 4 controls are analyzed, many control rules are relatively insensitive to moderate-sized errors. Yet, analytical runs have traditionally consisted of 2 to 4 controls.

Effective quality control procedures require sensitivity to both types of error and an acceptably low false rejection rate. Improved sensitivity to both random and systematic errors can be achieved by combining quality control rules. Quality control procedures using combinations of rules are called *"multirule control procedures"* or multirule procedures. Multirule procedures define both the rules and the order in which the rules are applied to the control data.

Multirule procedures, like control rules, can be applied within or across control materials. If a control procedure considers control observations from only 1 control material, then that procedure is used within control materials. If a procedure uses control observations from multiple control materials, then that procedure is used across control materials. Similarly, some procedures may be applied to control observations obtained within an analytical run or across analytical runs. Applying a control procedure within a run means that only control observations from that run are evaluated. Applying a control procedure across runs means that 1 or more control observations from 1 run are evaluated along with 1 or more control observations from the previous run or runs.

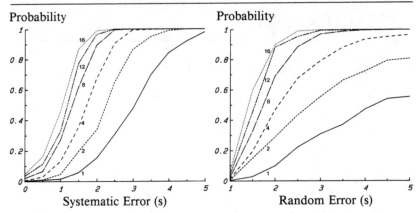

Figure 4–1 Power function curves for the $1_{3s}/2_{2s}$ control procedure. X-axis: size of error in standard deviations, Y-axis: probability of rejection, P_{ed} (P_{ed} = P_{fr} when systematic error is 0 or random error is 1).

EXAMPLES OF MULTIRULE CONTROL PROCEDURES

$1_{3s}/2_{2s}$

The simplest multirule procedure combines 2 rules, 1 with sensitivity to random error and 1 with sensitivity to systematic error. The $1_{3s}/2_{2s}$ combination rule is an example. For the 2_{2s} rule alone, with N = 2, the P_{ed} for a shift of 2s is 0.24 and the P_{ed} for a doubling of random error is 0.05. For the 1_{3s} rule with N = 2, the P_{ed} for a shift of 2s is 0.27, and the P_{ed} for a doubling of random error is 0.22. When the 1_{3s} and 2_{2s} rules are used together (ie, reject when either rule is violated) with N = 2, the P_{ed} for a shift of 2s is increased to 0.35, and the P_{ed} for a doubling of random error is increased to 0.28. These increases in the P_{ed} for both random and systematic errors represent approximately a 25% improvement over the P_{ed} for either rule used alone. The P_{fr} is still about 0.01. Power functions for the $1_{3s}/2_{2s}$ combination rule are shown in Figure 4–1.

$1_{3s}/2_{2s}/R_{4s}$ Control Procedure

For a small N, the P_{ed} for random error can be slightly improved by including the R_{4s} rule. The P_{ed} for a doubling of random error is somewhat increased from 0.28 for the $1_{3s}/2_{2s}$ rule to 0.31 for the $1_{3s}/2_{2s}/R_{4s}$ rule and 2 controls. The P_{fr} is about 0.02, which demonstrates that combining control rules increases the P_{fr} as well as the P_{ed}.

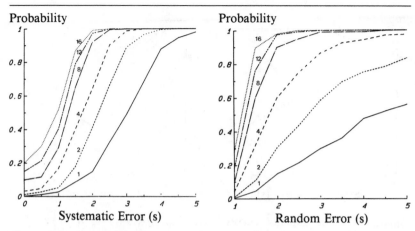

Figure 4-2 Power function curves for the $1_{3s}/2_{2s}/R_{4s}$ control procedure.

In this case the increase in the P_{ed} is greater than the increase in the P_{fr}, and the P_{fr} is still acceptably low. Power functions are given in Figure 4-2.

Haven recommended use of the $1_{3s}/2_{2s}/R_{4s}$ rule (although he did not express it in these terms) in 1974 and again in 1980.[1,2] He provided a step-by-step procedure, including plotting of control results. The procedure specifies that each run include 2 control materials of different concentrations. In this procedure, a run is rejected if 1 of 3 conditions is satisfied:

1. 1 control is more than 3s from its mean (1_{3s} rule applied).
2. Both controls are more than 2s from their respective means (2_{2s} and R_{4s} rule applied within run and across control materials).
3. On 2 successive runs 1 control material is more than 2s from its mean (2_{2s} and R_{4s} rule applied across runs and within materials).

It is fairly common to omit testing for condition 3, testing only for conditions 1 and 2, but this procedure omits control information from previous runs. When only 2 controls are analyzed, once each per run, and control information from the previous run is ignored, large errors at 1 control concentration can persist from run to run without being detected.

$1_{3s}/2_{2s}/R_{4s}/4_{1s}/10_{\bar{x}}$ Control Procedure

Westgard, et al recommended a combination of 5 rules, those suggested by Haven plus the 4_{1s} and $10_{\bar{x}}$ rules. This combination of rules,

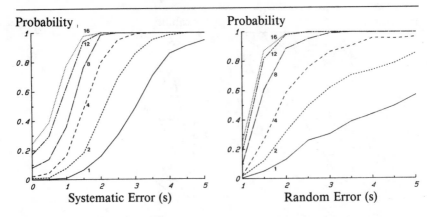

Figure 4–3   Power function curves for the $1_{3s}/2_{2s}/R_{4s}/4_{1s}/10_{\bar{x}}$ Westgard Multirule Shewhart Control Procedure.

$1_{3s}/2_{2s}/R_{4s}/4_{1s}/10_{\bar{x}}$ has become known as the Westgard multirule control procedure.[1,3] Power functions for the Westgard multirule are presented in Figure 4–3. Adding the 4_{1s} and $10_{\bar{x}}$ rules increases the P_{ed} for systematic error, although the systematic error must persist for at least 4 or 10 control observations, respectively, before these rules become effective. When there are 4 control observations within a run, the P_{ed} for a shift of 2s is increased from 0.66 for the $1_{3s}/2_{2s}/R_{4s}$ combination rule to 0.80 for the Westgard $1_{3s}/2_{2s}/R_{4s}/4_{1s}/10_{\bar{x}}$ multirule. Figure 4–3 also shows that smaller shifts are more likely to be detected.

When there are only 2 controls per run, the 4_{1s} and $10_{\bar{x}}$ rules cannot be used in the first run. By the end of the second run with 2 controls per run, the 4_{1s} control rule increases the P_{ed} of a 2s shift to 0.68, compared to 0.58, the P_{ed} for the $1_{3s}/2_{2s}/R_{4s}$ control procedure for 2 runs.

Westgard suggested a manual implementation of the multirule control procedure using 2 control charts, 1 for the low concentration material and the other for the high concentration material. This implementation is called the Westgard manual multirule Shewhart procedure. The control charts have lines which represent the mean and the following control limits: mean ± 1s, mean ± 2s, mean ± 3s. An example using a multirule control chart is presented in Exercise 4–1.

In the typical application of the Westgard multirule control procedure, an analytical run to be tested includes the high and low control materials. The suggested manual implementation differs from automated implementations in 2 respects, the 1_{2s} rule is used as a screening rule, and the R_{4s} rule is simplified. The laboratorian simply checks for violations of the 1_{2s} control rule; if there are none, the run is accepted. A violation of the 1_{2s} control rule is treated as a "warning" and is followed by inspection of the control data with the other control rules. Thus, unless the 1_{2s} rule is violated, it is not necessary to check for violations of the 1_{3s}, 2_{2s}, R_{4s}, 4_{1s}, or $10_{\bar{x}}$ rules. The R_{4s} rule is slightly modified; to violate the R_{4s} rule, successive control results must span the mean $\pm$ 2s range, which is more easily recognized on a quality control chart than a difference of 4s between successive control results. These 2 modifications greatly simplify the manual procedure and result in only a small loss of the P_{ed} as compared to a multirule application which uses no screening rule and the usual R_{4s} control rule.[3] In some computerized implementations of the procedure, use of the 1_{2s} rule as a screen is optional.

Because the Westgard multirule is widely practiced, we present a detailed description of the procedure. We have modified the original Westgard multirule in 2 ways. First, we have interchanged the order of the application of the 1_{3s} and the 2_{2s} control rules. Second, violations of the $10_{\bar{x}}$ control rule do not always require rejection of the analytical run; often the patient data may be reported with calibration-associated problems investigated afterward. (*We don't agree completely on this. GSC feels that runs should not be rejected for $10_{\bar{x}}$ failures. RNC feels that runs should be rejected for $10_{\bar{x}}$ failures across controls whenever shifts of less than 2s must be detected in order to maintain analytical errors within medically acceptable limits. If shifts up to 2s are medically acceptable, runs need not be rejected for $10_{\bar{x}}$ failures. The subject of medically tolerable errors is covered in Chapter 5.*) A schematic of the flow chart for implementing this procedure is shown in Figure 4–4. Whenever a run is accepted, the patient data can be reported. Whenever a run is rejected, patient data cannot be reported without the approval of the supervisor.

1. Analyze the 2 different control materials and record their results. Plot the control results on the appropriate control chart.

2. Test the control results with the 1_{2s} rule. *Accept* the run if both controls are within their mean $\pm$ 2s limits. If 1 or more control results exceed the mean $\pm$ 2s limits, do not report the patients' results. Inspect the control data further, using additional control rules.

3. Inspect the control data within the run.

    (a) Test the 2 control results with the 2_{2s} rule (across control ma-

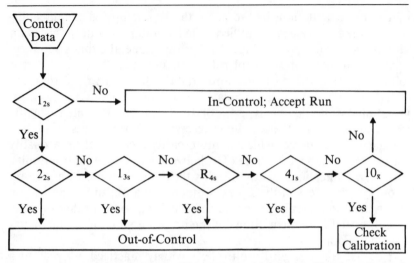

Figure 4–4 Flow chart of a modified Westgard Multirule Shewhart Control Procedure ($1_{3s}/2_{2s}/R_{4s}/4_{1s}/10_x$) using the 1_{2s} control screening rule.

terials) and *reject* the run if both control observations exceed the same mean ± 2s limits.

(b) Test with the 1_{3s} rule and *reject* the run if 1 control observation exceeds the mean ± 3s limits.

(c) Test the 2 control results with the R_{4s} rule (across control materials) and *reject* the run if 1 control result exceeds the mean + 2s limit and the other exceeds the mean − 2s limit.

4. Inspect control data across runs
   (a) Test with the 2_{2s} rule within the control materials and *reject* if the most recent 2 observations on the same control material exceed the same mean + 2s or mean − 2s control limit.
   (b) Test with the 4_{1s} rule across control materials and *reject* if the most recent 4 consecutive control observations exceed the same mean + 1s or mean − 1s limit.
   (c) Test with the 4_{1s} within control materials and *reject* if the most recent 4 control observations on the same control material exceed the same mean + 1s or mean − 1s limit.
   (d) Test with the 10_x rule across control materials. If the most recent 10 observations fall on the same side of the mean, report the patient data but check for correctable calibration or control-related problems (see comments above concerning 10_x rule).

(e) Test with the $10_{\bar{x}}$ rule within control materials. If the most recent 10 observations of the same control material fall on the same side of the mean, report the patient data but check for correctable calibration or control-related problems.

5. *Accept* the run when none of the rules indicates a lack of statistical control.

This procedure makes it clear that any 1_{2s} violation in the present run may require checking of the previous run(s) for continuing control problems. When a run is rejected, the control rule which is violated can indicate the error type. Random error is indicated by violations of the 1_{3s} and R_{4s} rules. Systematic error is indicated by the 2_{2s}, 4_{1s}, and $10_{\bar{x}}$, and if very large, the 1_{3s} rules. These hints as to the type of error are an aid to troubleshooting, although the 1_{3s} rule does respond to both random and systematic errors. However, there is 1 caveat: errors are often of mixed type. This assistance in determining the cause of an out-of-control run may be 1 reason for the popularity of this multi-rule procedure. Exercise 4–1 illustrates the application of the Westgard manual multirule procedure to typical control data.

A modification of the manual Westgard procedure in which the control data are charted in a tabular format is described in Chapter 9.

Other Multirule Procedures

The Haven and Westgard procedures are the most commonly used multirule control procedures. Some sources give substitutions which can be made to increase the P_{ed}: $1_{2.5s}$ or $1_{2.58s}$ for 1_{3s},[4] and $7_{\bar{x}}$, $8_{\bar{x}}$, $9_{\bar{x}}$, or $12_{\bar{x}}$ for $10_{\bar{x}}$.[5,6] These substitutions, however, may lead to dramatic increases in the P_{fr}, especially for a large N.

All of the multirule procedures discussed thus far are based on control rules in which single or groups of sequential control results are compared to control limits based on multiples of standard deviations from the mean. These control rules are termed "counting rules" because the number of consecutive controls which exceed the limit are counted. Counting rules are popular because they are easily implemented without a computer. The rules which are described in the following sections rely on testing a statistic of the control data as a group (mean, range, etc) rather than testing the actual data.

Mean and Range; Mean and Chi-square Rules

Mean and range rules can be combined to provide a very high P_{ed} with a low P_{fr} when 4 or more observations are available. Power func-

EXERCISE 4-1 Illustration of use of the multirule procedure to interpret control data. Two controls are run daily for a glucose procedure. Data are plotted on quality control charts, as described in Chapter 3. Apply the Westgard multirule procedure to the data, interpreting the control charts for both controls to determine the days on which a violation of the screening rule occurs, the action to be taken on each of these days, and the most likely kind of error (for rejected runs).

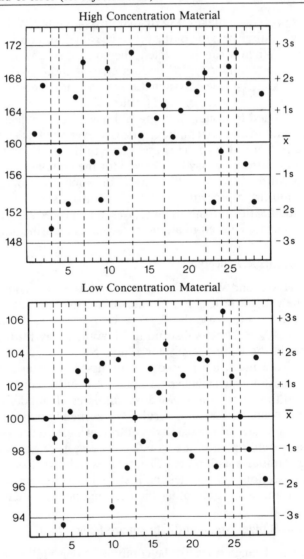

ANSWER:

Day	Control	Rule Violation
day 3	high	1_{2s}, warning; accept run
day 4	low	1_{3s}, reject run, random or systematic
day 7	low and high	4_{1s} across controls, across runs; reject run, systematic
day 10	low and high	R_{4s} across controls; reject run, random
day 13	high	1_{2s}, warning, accept run
day 17	low	1_{2s}, warning, accept run
day 22	high	$10_{\bar{x}}$ within control, across runs; reject run, systematic
day 24	low	1_{3s}, reject run, random or systematic
day 25	high	1_{2s}, warning, accept run
day 26	high	2_{2s} within control, across runs; reject run, systematic

tions for $\bar{X}_{0.01}/R_{0.01}$ are given in Figure 4–5. With N = 4, the P_{ed} for a shift of 2s is 0.90, and the P_{ed} for a doubling of random error is 0.72, while the P_{fr} is only 0.02. When N = 8, the P_{ed} increases to virtually 1.00 for a shift of 2s, and to 0.85 for a doubling of random error. The P_{fr} is constant. The combination $\bar{X}_{0.05}/R_{0.05}$ is extremely sensitive to error, but cannot be recommended because of its high P_{fr} of 0.10. For N ≤ 4, multirule combinations using counting rules perform as well as, or better than, the combination $\bar{X}_{0.05}/R_{0.05}$. With a large N, mean/range combinations can detect very small errors, and combinations like $\bar{X}_{0.01}/R_{0.01}$ can be used to provide a lower P_{fr} with good sensitivity to systematic error.

The principal disadvantage of mean and range rules is that the same number of replicate determinations of the same control material must be made in each run. Also, the performance of mean rules may be affected by large between-run components of variance. These effects will be demonstrated in Chapter 6.

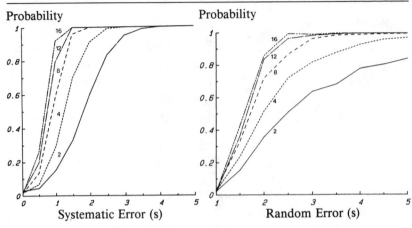

Figure 4–5 Power function curves for $\bar{X}_{0.01}/R_{0.01}$ control procedure.

Precision/Accuracy Trend Analysis

Trend analysis can provide error detection similar to that of mean and range rules, without the requirement of mean and range rules to test the control data in batches. Combination precision/accuracy trend analysis permits assessment of each control result for precision and accuracy trends as it is received; however, the repeated testing significantly increases the P_{fr}.[7] In practice, limits must be calculated at reduced sensitivity for error detection in order to limit the P_{fr}. Trend analysis has not previously been used to its full potential because it requires computerization for practical use; computerization is now available to utilize trend analysis efficiently. Cembrowski et al have applied trend analysis to quality control of continuous-flow analyzers.[8] More recently, Douville, Cembrowski, and Strauss have applied an optimized exponential smoothing technique to the quality control of endocrine assays.[9]

Cumulative Sum/Multirule Procedures

Cumulative sum procedures have been widely used in industry, but have not been well accepted in the clinical laboratory, presumably because of computational difficulty, and because of the complex relationship of the cumulative sum to the size of the analytical error. With the advent of computerized quality control, cumulative sum procedures are now more easily implemented. Cumulative sum procedures

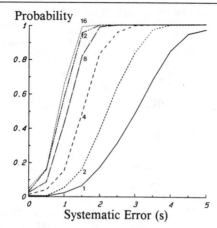

Figure 4–6 Power function curves for the $CS^{1.0s}_{2.7s}/1_{3s}$ control procedure.

do not require that the number of controls per run be constant, and can be used to test individual control data as they are produced. There is no rule for random error which is exactly analogous to cusum; cumulative sum may be combined with 1_{3s} and/or R_{4s}, or precision trend analysis rules to detect random error. Figure 4–6 shows the performance characteristics of the $1_{3s}/CS^{1.0s}_{2.7s}$ control procedure for the detection of systematic error. The $1_{3s}/CS^{1.0s}_{2.7s}$ combination has a higher P_{ed} for systematic error than the $1_{3s}/2_{2s}/R_{4s}/4_{1s}/10_{\bar{x}}$ combination, and has a lower P_{fr} as the N increases. The performance characteristics of the $1_{3s}/CS^{1.0s}_{2.7s}$ combination for the detection of random error are roughly equivalent to those of the 1_{3s} control. Comparing the $1_{3s}/CS^{1.0s}_{2.7s}$ to mean/range rules, for equal numbers of control observations, the combination $\bar{X}_{0.01}/R_{0.01}$ is superior, having a higher P_{ed} and a lower P_{fr}, especially with an increasing N.

Preferred Control Procedures for Various N

Recommendations made by Westgard and the authors for selecting combinations of rules for various N's are summarized in Table 4–1. Rule selection depends on the size of error which must be detected to maintain the fitness of patient testing results for medical use, and on the frequency of false rejections which can be tolerated; Table 4–1 is intended to provide a starting point from which the reader can optimize quality control rules for his or her own particular use.

Table 4-1 Multirule combinations for different numbers of controls included in run.

| N | Recommended control rules | |
	Individual runs	Consecutive runs
1	1_{2s}	4_{1s}
2	$1_{3s}/2_{2s}/R_{4s}$ $1_{2.5s}$	$4_{1s}/10_{\bar{x}}$ or $12_{\bar{x}}$
3	$1_{3s}/(2 \text{ of } 3)_{2s}/R_{4s}$ $1_{2.5s}$	$9_{\bar{x}}$ or $12_{\bar{x}}$
4	$1_{3s}/2_{2s}/R_{4s}/4_{1s}$	$8_{\bar{x}}$ or $12_{\bar{x}}$
6	$1_{3s}/2_{2s}/R_{0.01}/4_{1s}$ $1_{3s}/(3 \text{ of } 6)_{2s}$	$12_{\bar{x}}$
4–10	Mean/range $1_{3s}/(m \text{ of } n)_{2s}$	Trend analysis, Cumulative Sum
4–20	Mean/range	Trend analysis, Cumulative Sum

Note: When R_{4s} is used above with $N > 2$, R_{4s} is violated whenever the range between *any* 2 of the controls exceeds 4s.

Modified with permission. From Westgard JO, Barry PL, Hunt MR, Groth T: A multirule Shewhard chart for quality control in clinical chemistry. Clin Chem 27:493–501, 1981. And from Westgard JO, Barry PL: Cost-effective quality control: managing the quality and productivity of analytical processes. AACC Press, Washington, DC, 1986, pp 118–137.

When only one control is analyzed per run, the 1_{2s} rule should be applied to the individual control results. The 4_{1s} rule helps detect systematic error which persists over several runs.

When there are 2 controls per run, either the $1_{3s}/2_{2s}/R_{4s}$ rules or the $1_{2.5s}$ rule can be applied to control results within the run, and the 4_{1s} and $10_{\bar{x}}$ or $12_{\bar{x}}$ rules are applied across runs.

Three different control materials are often used in each run in blood gas analysis and immunoassays in order to check performance in 3 different concentration ranges. When there are 3 control results per run, the 2_{2s} rule is modified to reject whenever 2 of the 3 controls exceed the same mean $\pm$ 2s limit, and called the $(2 \text{ of } 3)_{2s}$ rule. This is the most common proportion rule. Similarly, the R_{4s} rule is modified to reject whenever 2 of the 3 controls exceed opposite mean $\pm$ 2s limits (at least 1 control value exceeding the mean + 2s limit and at least 1 control value exceeding the mean − 2s limit). Consecutive runs are monitored by use of either the $9_{\bar{x}}$ or $12_{\bar{x}}$ rule. For $N = 3$, the P_{ed} for detecting a shift of 2s in 1 run is 0.63 and the P_{ed} for a doubling of random error is 0.43. Alternatively, the $1_{2.5s}$ rule may be used to judge an individual run, with virtually the same sensitivity to error.

When there are 4 controls per run the $1_{3s}/2_{2s}/R_{4s}/4_{1s}$ rule is used to judge the acceptability of the individual run, and either the $8_{\bar{x}}$ or $12_{\bar{x}}$ rule is used to signal the presence of small, but correctable, persistent shifts. For less than 5 control observations, the Westgard multirule control procedures using the simple counting rules and the $1_{2.5s}$ rule are generally preferred because they perform approximately as well as the more complicated rules, and can be used across controls as well as with a variable number of controls. For 5 or more control observations, the P_{fr} for these rules becomes excessive. However, appropriately selected proportion rules, $(m \text{ of } n)_{ks}$, are still effective.

Mean/range combination rules can be used efficiently for judging individual runs with large numbers of controls. Trend analysis and cumulative sum may be used to monitor consecutive runs.

PREDICTIVE VALUES OF DECISIONS TO ACCEPT OR REJECT ANALYTICAL RUNS

The selection of a control procedure for an analytical method involves a compromise between an acceptable false rejection rate and adequate sensitivity to medically significant errors. If a control procedure's ability to detect medically significant errors is too low, and analytical error is present, subsequent test results will not be fit for medical use, even though the method may appear to be in control. If the control procedure's P_{fr} is too high, there will be a high proportion of runs which are rejected and repeated but without any significant change in measured concentrations. A tenuous relationship between a rejection signal and an identifiable source of error will result in a loss of confidence in the control procedure.

The performance of a quality control procedure can be further described by the same predictive value terms used to describe the performance of a diagnostic test.[10] Westgard has calculated 2 predictive value terms for quality control tests: the predictive value of a reject signal, PV_r, analogous to the predictive value of a positive test, and the predictive value of an accept signal, PV_a, analogous to the predictive value of a negative test.[11,12] Ideally, the predictive value should be 1.00 or 100%. The PV_r is the proportion of all reject signals which are truly indicative of analytical error. If there are 100 runs in which a quality control procedure has indicated an error, but error was present in only 50 of these runs, then the PV_r is 50/100 or 0.50. The PV_a is the proportion of all accept signals which are error free. For example,

Table 4-2 Predictive value characteristics of accept/reject decisions

Analytical Runs	Reject Decision	Accept Decision
With errors	$n_{tr} = n(prevP_{ed})$	$n_{fa} = n(1 - P_{ed})$
Without errors	$n_{fr} = n(1 - prev)P_{fr}$	$n_{ta} = n(1 - prev)(1 - P_{fr})$

$$PV_r = \frac{n_{tr}}{n_{tr} + n_{fr}} = \frac{prevP_{ed}}{prevP_{ed} + (1 - prev)P_{fr}}$$

$$PV_a = \frac{n_{ta}}{n_{ta} + n_{fa}} = \frac{(1 - prev)(1 - P_{fr})}{(1 - prev)(1 - P_{fr}) + prev(1 - P_{ed})}$$

Modified with permission. From Westgard JO, Groth T: A predictive value model for quality control: effects of the prevalence of errors on the performance of control procedures. Am J Clin Pathol 80:49–56, 1983.

Note: Based on the P_{fr}, P_{ed}, and prevalence of errors (prev). Prevalence is expressed as a decimal fraction. Of a total of n runs, the number of runs rejected with errors is n_{tr}, and the number rejected without errors is n_{fr}. The PV_r is predictive value of a reject decision and the PV_a is predictive value of an accept decision.

if there were 100 runs which were accepted because a quality control procedure indicated the lack of error, but error was present in 5 of these runs (95 error-free runs), the PV_a would be 95/100 or 0.95. The predictive value of an accept or reject decision depends on the prevalence of error.

Westgard has combined the prevalence of analytical errors with the P_{ed} and the P_{fr} of specific quality control rules and has derived the PV_r and PV_a for various prevalences of error. The equations for calculating these predictive values are summarized in Table 4–2. The PV_r can be increased by decreasing the P_{fr}, or by increasing the P_{ed}. The PV_r increases with increasing prevalence (prev). These relationships are demonstrated in Figure 4–7. The PV_r is much higher at low prevalence (prev = 0.01) for multirule, 1_{3s} and $\bar{X}_{0.01}$ than it is for the 1_{2s} rule, since the P_{fr} is much higher for the 1_{2s} rule. As prevalence increases, the difference in PV_r caused by the P_{fr} is less striking.

The PV_a can be increased by increasing the P_{ed}. It is less sensitive to increases in the P_{fr}. The PV_a decreases as prevalence increases. Figure 4–8 demonstrates these relationships, showing the dependence of the PV_a on the P_{ed} and prev.

The relevance of the relationships described above may be shown by an example. Consider the predictive value of run acceptance decisions for an analytical method whose prevalence of significant systematic errors (those shifts exceeding 2s) is 2% (0.02). Assume there

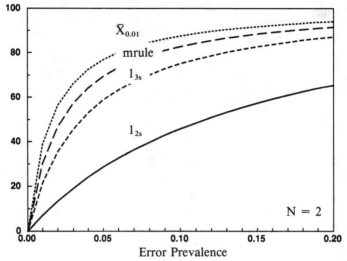

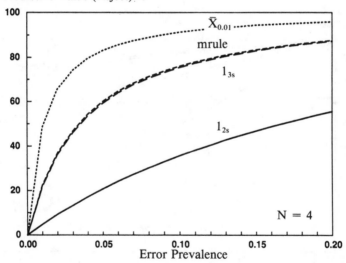

Figure 4–7 Relationship of the PV_r to error prevalence for various control procedures employing 2 and 4 controls. A shift of 2s is being considered. (For 2 controls, mrule = Westgard multirule: $P_{fr} = 0.01$, $P_{ed} = 0.43$; 1_{2s}: $P_{fr} = 0.10$, $P_{ed} = 0.76$; 1_{3s}: $P_{fr} = 0.01$, $P_{ed} = 0.27$; $\bar{X}_{0.01}$: $P_{fr} = 0.01$, $P_{ed} = 0.76$. For 4 controls, mrule: $P_{fr} = 0.03$, $P_{ed} = 0.83$; 1_{2s}: $P_{fr} = 0.19$, $P_{ed} = 0.95$; 1_{3s}: $P_{fr} = 0.02$, $P_{ed} = 0.57$; $\bar{X}_{0.01}$: $P_{fr} = 0.01$, $P_{ed} = 0.93$.)

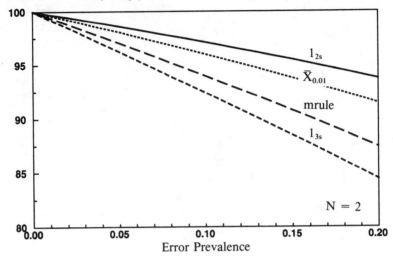

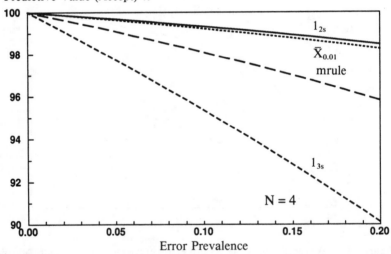

Figure 4-8   Relationship of the PV_a to error prevalence for various control procedures employing 2 and 4 controls. A shift of 2s is being considered. (mrule = Westgard multirule: $P_{fr} = 0.01$, $P_{ed} = 0.43$; 1_{2s}: $P_{fr} = 0.10$, $P_{ed} = 0.76$; 1_{3s}: $P_{fr} = 0.01$, $P_{ed} = 0.27$; $x_{0.01}$: $P_{fr} = 0.10$, $P_{ed} = 0.76$. See Figure 4-7 legend for data.)

are 2 controls per run. If the 1_{2s} rule is used as the criterion for run acceptance decisions, the P_{fr} is 0.10, and the P_{ed} is 0.76. The predictive value of a reject decision (PV_r) is 0.13, which is to say that only 13% of rejected runs will really have large errors. Eighty seven percent of rejected runs will be false rejections. If the Westgard multirule procedure is used instead, the P_{fr} is 0.01, the P_{ed} is 0.43, and the PV_r is increased to 0.47. The PV_r increases with decreasing P_{fr}, increasing P_{ed}, and increasing prevalence.

For the same method (error prevalence of 0.02), the predictive value of an accept decision (PV_a) using the 1_{2s} rule is 0.995. Using the Westgard multirule, the PV_a is 0.988. The PV_a increases with decreasing prevalence and increasing P_{ed}. The PV_a responds most strongly to the prevalence and the P_{ed}, but it also increases with decreasing P_{fr}, although not as much as the PV_r.

PREVALENCE OF ANALYTIC ERRORS

It is impossible to determine the prevalence of all analytic errors whose magnitudes exceed the inherent random error of a method because errors which slightly exceed the inherent error are effectively indistinguishable from the inherent random error. It is easier to measure the prevalence of errors which are much larger than inherent error. Thus, the observed prevalence of errors is likely to underestimate the true prevalence.

A thorough study of prevalence of analytical error in current blood gas instrumentation was done by Metzger et al, who investigated the efficacy of duplicate analysis of blood gas specimens on separate blood gas analyzers.[13] In their study of duplicate analyses of over 1500 specimens, they found overall error prevalences between 0.6% and 3.2% for an older model blood gas analyzer (Corning Model 175, Corning Medical, Medfield, MA) and prevalences between 0.0% and 0.9% for a state-of-the-art (1986) blood gas analyzer (Corning Model 178). While overall prevalences of error were low, there were periods during the study when error rates reached 16% for the older analyzer and 6% for the newer model. Details of the design of the study are given in the report by Metzger et al.[13]

Error prevalences have also been studied in the area of coagulation testing, where the means of duplicate tests are usually reported. In a study assessing the need for duplicate analysis for prothrombin time (PT) and activated partial thromboplastin time (aPTT) assays, Foucar and Nymeyer[14] found an overall error prevalence of approximately 1.6%. Cornelison et al[15] reported an error prevalence of approximately

0.2% for PT testing. Scheer et al[16] and Keshgegian et al[17] reported error prevalences of less than 1% and 2% for PT and aPTT, respectively.

Blaabjerg et al studied the prevalence of errors in a manual triio-dothyronine radioimmunoassay procedure and reported a prevalence of 7%.[18] In a study of errors on an automated system, Jorgensen, et al found a prevalence of 13% in calcium analysis by the o-cresol-phthalein complexone method on an automated chemistry analyzer.[19] Aronsson and Groth studied error frequencies for multiple analytical methods on 3 automated multichannel analyzers.[20] In their initial check procedure (startup quality control check), they found prevalences varying from 0% to 40%. In monitoring single runs after startup, the prevalences ranged from 0% to 25%. Long-term assessment demonstrated a prevalence of between 0% and 4%.

From our own experiences it seems that the prevalence of error for most methods is low, around 1% to 2%, but most laboratories have at least 1 method which is especially troublesome and has an error prevalence exceeding 10%.

RESPONSE TO CONTROL RULE VIOLATIONS

For years it was common practice to include at least 2 control samples in an analytical run, and to repeat any run with a 1_{2s} control rule violation. With a low prevalence of errors, the rejection was most often a false rejection. When a multirule procedure is used instead of 1_{2s} control rules, both the P_{fr} and the P_{ed} are reduced with the P_{fr} reduced proportionally more than the P_{ed}. Figure 4–7 shows that violations of multirule procedures are more likely to be caused by real errors (higher PV_r). Merely repeating the controls or even the entire analytical run is not an acceptable corrective action. The P_{ed} of the Westgard multirule is relatively low, eg, on the order of 0.43 for a shift of 2s. On the average, more than 2 analytical runs would be required (or analyzing 4 or more controls) to incur another rejection due to a shift of 2s. Therefore, troubleshooting must take place before the run is repeated. Extra control replicates should be included in the repeat run in order to increase the P_{ed}. The increase in the P_{fr} caused by the extra controls is justified by the need for an increased P_{ed} when an error is suspected. Again, it should be pointed out that the rule violated helps identify the type of error, and promotes more effective trouble-shooting.

Because extra control replicates are included in the repeat run, it is not necessary to combine control data from the rejected run with the new control data. The repeat run should stand alone and should not be grouped with prior data for run acceptance decisions. Any future consideration of the data from the rejected run is only for retrospective analysis of frequency of control failures (eg with proportion rules) or to determine the presence of a trend. Data from a rejected run should not be included in calculations of the mean and standard deviation for purposes of control range calculations.

Infrequently, demands for rapid turnaround of patient results may require consideration of result reporting despite control rule violations which would normally lead to run rejection. In an actual case, an emergency room patient's glucose was measured at 295 mg/dL, but both controls (means and standard deviations are approximately 70 and 2 mg/dL, and 260 and 4 mg/dL, respectively) were repeatedly between 2s and 3s from their means. The backup method was not operative and a minimum of 45 minutes would have been required to completely troubleshoot the glucose method. In this situation, the observed systematic error was judged to be insufficient to invalidate the medical usefulness of the patient result and the 295 mg/dL result was reported. Such decisions should be made at the supervisor/pathologist level on a case-by-case basis, but the analyst should be able to evaluate the type and magnitude of the error through careful interpretation of the control data.

MULTISTAGE CONTROL PROCEDURES

Quality control procedures can be customized to complement the performance characteristics of automated analytical systems.[20] When errors occur in systems which process samples in batches, they often are detectable at startup if the control procedure is sufficiently sensitive. Thus, high sensitivity to errors is desirable during startup, even if the P_{fr} must be relatively high in order to achieve sensitivity. If no errors are detected, and the analytical procedure is stable, a less sensitive procedure can be used to monitor performance during the remainder of the run.

For retrospective analysis, rules relying on a large N may be used to detect small errors (for example, comparison of monthly means and standard deviations with previously established means and standard deviations). Retrospective analysis helps detect the need for improved maintenance and training. Specific multistage quality control procedures will be reviewed in Chapter 8.

REFERENCES

1. Haven GT: Outline for quality control decisions. Pathologist 28:373-378, 1974.

2. Haven GT, Larson NS, and Ross JW: Quality control outline: 1980. Pathologist 34:619-622, 1980.

3. Westgard JO, Barry PL, Hunt MR, Groth T: A multirule Shewhart chart for quality control in clinical chemistry. Clin Chem 27:493-501, 1981.

4. Blum AS: Computer evaluation of statistical procedures, and a new quality-control statistical procedure. Clin Chem 31:206-212, 1985.

5. Westgard JO and Groth T: Power functions for statistical control rules. Clin Chem 25:863-869, 1979.

6. Westgard JO, Groth T, Aronsson T, et al: Performance characteristics of rules for internal quality control: Probabilities for false rejection and error detection. Clin Chem 23:1857-1867, 1977.

7. Westgard JO, Groth T: Design and evaluation of statistical control procedures: applications of a computer "quality control simulator" program. Clin Chem 27:1536-1545, 1981.

8. Cembrowski GS, Westgard JO, Eggert AA, Toren EC, Jr: Trend detection in control data: optimization and interpretation of Trigg's technique for trend analysis. Clin Chem 21:1396-1405, 1975.

9. Douville P, Cembrowski GS, and Strauss J: Evaluation of the average of patients, application to endocrine assays. Clin Chim Acta 167:173-185, 1987.

10. Galen RS, Gambino RS: Beyond normality: the predictive value and efficiency of medical diagnoses. John Wiley & Sons, New York, 1975.

11. Westgard JO, Groth T: A predictive value model for quality control: effects of the prevalence of errors on the performance of control procedures. Am J Clin Pathol 80:49-56, 1983.

12. Westgard JO, Barry PL: Cost-effective quality control: managing the quality and productivity of analytical processes. AACC Press, Washington, DC, 1986, pp 118-137.

13. Metzger LF, Stauffer WB, Krupinski AV, et al: Detecting errors in blood-gas measurements by analysis with two instruments. Clin Chem 33:512-517, 1987.

14. Foucar K, Nymeyer V: To replicate or not to replicate, that was the question. Am J Clin Pathol 84:407, 1985.

15. Cornelison GS, Rollins A, Santoro, SA: Duplicate coagulation assays warranted. Am J Clin Pathol 84:261-262,1985.

16. Scheer WD, Catrou PG, Lipscomb GE, Boudreau DA: A comprehensive evaluation of the performance of duplicate prothrombin time and activated partial thromboplastin time assays. Am J Clin Pathol 85:456-462,1986.

17. Keshgegian AA, Mann JM, Cooper JH: Is duplicate testing for prothrombin time and activated partial thrombo-plastin time necessary? Arch Pathol Lab Med 110:520-522,1986.

18. Blaabjerg O, Hyltoft Petersen P, Dreyer T, et al: The impact of quality control materials on the performance of an internal quality control system: 3. Experiences from s-triiodothyronine analysis. Scan J Clin Lab Invest 44 (suppl 172):79-86, 1984.

19. Jorgensen PJ, Horder M, Blaabjerg O, et al: The impact of quality control materials on the performance of an internal quality control system: 2. Experiences from s-calcium analysis. Scand J Clin Lab Invest 44 (suppl 172):71-77, 1984.

20. Aronsson T, Groth T: Nested control procedures for internal analytical quality control. Theoretical design and practical evaluation. Scand J Clin Lab Invest 44 (suppl 172):51–64, 1984.

CHAPTER FIVE

Medical Usefulness Requirements of Analytical Systems

Ten to twenty years ago, there was an obvious trend toward developing new analyzers with improved precision and accuracy. The emergence of enzymatic methods greatly improved the precision and accuracy of analytes such as glucose, urea, and uric acid. Interferences were minimized with dialysis techniques. There was an awareness, both in the laboratory and in industry, that these improvements were necessary; cost was frequently a secondary issue. Recently there has been an influx of new analytical methods and instrumentation, some of which promote convenience or low cost at the expense of accuracy and precision. Instrument and method selection is now a tradeoff, so the following question must frequently be asked: "What is the maximum analytical inaccuracy and imprecision that can be tolerated for a specific test?"

Various approaches have been used to define standards for maximum allowable analytical error, including surveys, studies of interindividual and intraindividual variation, and even using the performance of state of the art analyzers as target values. These standards for allowable analytical error are important because they can be used by instrument manufacturers to establish guidelines for instrument performance, and also because they can be used to derive the performance required of quality control procedures.

This chapter is concerned with determining the error detection capability required of quality control procedures to guarantee the detection of unacceptably large errors. To make these estimates, 2 pieces of information are required: the performance standard, a statement of the maximum error that is medically allowable for the analyte, and the actual baseline performance characteristics of the analytical method to be controlled.

Two main sections divide this chapter. The first section compares the approaches used to derive performance standards for medically allowable analytical error. The second section is concerned with the transformation of the performance standard and a method's inherent analytical error into maximally allowable random or systematic error. In this section the inherent performance of 2 representative automated chemistry analyzers is transformed into maximum allowable random and systematic error. Chapter 8 will describe how the magnitudes of these maximum allowable errors can be used to select optimal quality control procedures.

ESTIMATION OF MAXIMUM ALLOWABLE ERROR

Physician and Laboratorian Survey

The most popular approach to the derivation of performance standards for maximum allowable error is the survey of clinicians and laboratorians. Barnett was one of the first to compile a list of medically allowable errors based on the synthesis of opinions of clinicians and laboratory specialists.[1] Although Barnett's list is over 20 years old, it is reproduced in Table 5-1 because we feel that Barnett's goals are minimum goals to achieve, ie, an analyzer should not exhibit a standard deviation higher than the allowable standard deviation(s) at the specified decision level concentrations. Also presented in Table 5-1 are the average monthly coefficients of variation (CVs) of 2 highly precise analyzers, the Dupont aca and the Kodak Ektachem 700. Even when analyzed on these 2 "state of the art" analyzers, at least 3 analytes, calcium, total carbon dioxide, and sodium, exhibit CVs which are close to the maximally acceptable CVs.

After Barnett's 1968 paper, more formal interview techniques were used to obtain estimates of allowable error. Brief clinical problems were usually presented with the interviewee asked to select test result values which were significantly different from an initial value. Two representative clinical problems follow:

Clinical Problem 5-1

The patient is a well-controlled diabetic in the hospital with a myocardial infarction. The laboratory reports a fasting plasma glucose level of 100 mg/dL. The test is reordered the next day. Which of the following indicates a clinically important change, ie, the value that alters the diagnosis or treatment or prompts further evaluation of the patient's condition? 115, 120, 125, 130, 135, 140, 145 mg/dL (Derived from Skendzel[2]).

Table 5-1   Allowable errors of various chemistry analytes.

Analyte	Decision Level	Allowable s	Allowable CV(%)	aca CV(%)	E-700 CV(%)
Albumin, g/dL	3.5	0.25	7.1	1.8	2.7
Bilirubin, mg/dL	1.0	0.2	20.0	7.8	10.7
Bilirubin, mg/dL	20.0	1.5	7.5		
Calcium, mg/dL	11.0	0.25	2.3	1.1	1.8
Chloride, mmol/L	90	2.0	2.2	1.3	1.0
Chloride, mmol/L	110	2.0	1.8	1.3	1.1
Cholesterol, mg/dL	240	7.20	3.0	1.4	2.0
CO_2, mmol/L	20	1.0	5.0	3.2	4.2
CO_2, mmol/L	30	1.0	3.3	3.8	4.6
Glucose, mg/dL	50	5.0	10.0	1.7	1.9
Glucose, mg/dL	100	5.0	5.0	2.0	1.2
Phosphorous, mg/dL	4.5	0.25	5.6	2.8	2.2
Potassium, mmol/L	3	0.25	8.3	1.5	1.5
Potassium, mmol/L	6	0.25	4.2	1.1	1.5
Sodium, mmol/L	150	2.0	1.3	0.9	1.1
Sodium, mmol/L	130	2.0	1.5	0.6	0.9
Total protein, g/dL	7.0	0.3	4.3	1.5	1.9
Urea nitrogen, mg/dL	27	2.0	7.4	2.7	3.7
Uric acid, mg/dL	6.0	0.5	8.3	1.6	1.7

Modified with permission. From Cembrowski GS. Analytical requirements for clinical chemistry. In: Quality assurance in physician office, bedside and home testing. Howanitz PJ, ed, College of American Pathologists, Skokie, IL, 1986, pp 160-163.

Note: Errors (expressed as s and CV) compared to the CVs of 2 representative (and highly precise) clinical chemistry analyzers—the Dupont aca (EI Dupont deNemours & Co, Wilmington, DE) and the Ektachem 700 (Eastman Kodak, Rochester, NY). CVs were obtained from average monthly standard deviations of multiple analyzers. The allowable errors are those of Barnett.[1] The clinically allowable error (E_a) can be computed from 2 × allowable s. Allowable error for cholesterol is from the recommendation of the Laboratory Standardization Panel of the National Cholesterol Education Program.[19]

CLINICAL PROBLEM 5-2

Internal abdominal injuries are suspected in a 6-year old child involved in an automobile accident. On admission, the hemoglobin is 13.0 g/dL. The test is repeated 2 hours later. Circle the value that would prompt you to investigate whether bleeding has occurred: 12.8, 12.6, 12.4, 12.2, 12.0, 11.8, 11.6, 11.4, 11.2, 11.0, 10.8, 10.6, 10.4, 10.2, 10.0 or lower (Derived from Skendzel et al[3]).

The results of these clinical problems can be very divergent and depend on the physician group interviewed. For this reason, the mode or median of the responses usually defines the maximum (or minimum) allowable value which is still clinically acceptable and does not need to be followed by any further action, including reordering the test or ordering followup tests. The difference between the initial value and maximum (or minimum) allowable value yields the maximum allowable error which is then transformed into a maximum allowable standard deviation.

Two histograms are shown in Figure 5-1, one representing the actual answers to Clinical Problem 5-2 from 83 pediatricians, and the other representing the theoretical distribution of hemoglobins about the original mean, 13.0 g/dL, which would be obtained from multiple hemoglobin determinations on a modern multichannel hematology analyzer. The actual median of the answers for Clinical Problem 5-2 was 11.6 g/dL. One half of the clinicians interviewed would not act until the level of the hemoglobin dropped to 11.6 g/dL or less. The maximum allowable error thus corresponds to the difference between the original concentration and the median survey value and is 13.0 − 11.6 g/dL or 1.4 g/dL. The maximum allowable error for hemoglobin, 1.4 g/dL, is then divided by a conversion factor to yield a maximum allowable standard deviation, which in turn can be transformed into a CV. This conversion factor used by various authors to convert maximum allowable error to a standard deviation has ranged from 2.3 to 2.8. For serial measurements, Skendzel et al divided the maximum allowable errors by 2.33. The maximum acceptable standard deviation would thus be 1.4/2.33, or 0.60 g/dL, which corresponds to an allowable CV of 4.9%. Figure 5-1 indicates that a large amount of error can be tolerated in the second hemoglobin measurement before it results in a hemoglobin value which is less than 11.6 g/dL. This maximum allowable standard deviation is approximately 4 times greater than the typical analytical standard deviation obtained for hemoglobin by modern multichannel hematology analyzers.

One of the most important assumptions in these studies is that the maximum allowable error is due strictly to analytical error. While physiologic variation and the effects of therapeutic intervention can account for part of the maximum allowable error, they are not considered. It is highly probable that the patient in Clinical Problem 5-2 is being given intravenous fluids which may result in hemodilution and a decreased hemoglobin. Unfortunately, dividing the maximum

Frequency

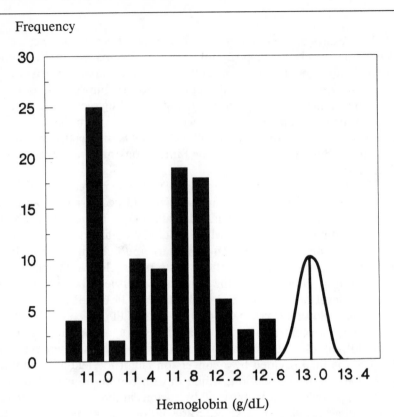

Hemoglobin (g/dL)

Figure 5–1   Results of survey of pediatricians' responses to Clinical Problem 5–2. The frequency histogram shows percentage of answers versus the minimum allowable hemoglobin that would result in further workup of the patient. Superimposed on the frequency histogram is the theoretical distribution of hemoglobin determinations analyzed on a modern multichannel analyzer (mean = 13.0, s = 0.12 g/dL).

(Survey data courtesy of LP Skendzel)

allowable error by a factor to derive the allowable standard deviation and ignoring therapy are necessary oversimplifications.

Probably the most comprehensive study to determine allowable error was that of Elion-Gerritzen[4] who personally interviewed 63 senior internal medicine specialists from four different countries. Her work was divided into 2 major sections. She first posed initial analyte values in the near abnormal range and then asked for a second value which would signal a significant change. Her values of maximum allowable

CVs are extremely close to those proposed by Barnett approximately 10 years earlier. In the second part of her study she solicited reference range limits and their corresponding action limits (values which would prompt clinician action including repeating the test or doing additional testing). With this technique she obtained maximum allowable CVs for both the lower and upper action limits. Elion-Gerritzen found that the normal range limit exactly matched the action limit for many of the tests. The implication of this finding is that *there are certain tests for which clinician behavior cannot tolerate error, either analytic or physiologic, about their reference levels*. Those tests and reference levels were: alkaline phosphatase, upper limit (UL); calcium, UL; cholesterol, UL; creatinine, UL; glucose, UL and lower limit (LL); phosphate, LL; total protein, UL; urea nitrogen, LL. Elion-Gerritzen's finding is particularly disconcerting for instrument designers!

Other investigators, including Campbell and Owen,[5] Skendzel,[2] Barrett et al,[6] and Skendzel, Barnett and Platt,[3] have used survey techniques to derive estimates of maximum allowable analytical error for clinical chemistry tests. Because of the variation in their research methodologies and the subjects surveyed, there are considerable differences in their findings.

Figure 5–2 summarizes the maximum allowable CVs of common chemistry analytes, as well as hemoglobin, and compares them to those obtained by Barnett,[1] Elion-Gerritzen,[4] and others. The graphical format highlights the lack of agreement on medically allowable CVs.

Little work has been done in surveying clinicians to establish maximum allowable errors for hematology tests. Figure 5–2 shows the maximum allowable CVs for hemoglobin. The reader is referred to the work of Skendzel, Barnett, and Platt, who determined error limits for hematocrit, hemoglobin, white cell count, mean corpuscular volume, and prothrombin time.[3] Shephard, Penberthy, and Fraser have used a survey approach to determine analytical goals for quantitative urine analytes, including sodium potassium, urea, creatinine, and calcium.[7]

Physiologic Variation

Laboratory tests are ordered for one of two principal purposes: (1) to rule out or confirm disease, in which an individual's laboratory results are compared to either a population reference range or the individual's reference range, and (2) to monitor therapy, in which serial determinations are made and compared to one another. The precision required to measure an analyte depends on how tightly its concentration is controlled, both within a population (interindividual variation)

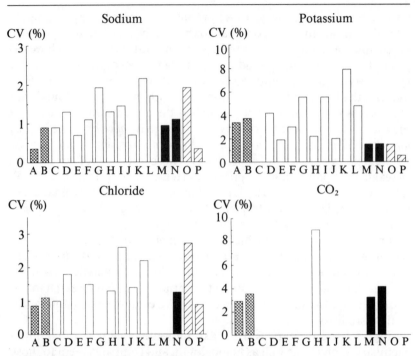

Figure 5-2 Estimates of maximum allowable analytical error for common clinical chemistry analytes and hemoglobin. The allowable analytical error is expressed as a coefficient of variation (CV). The cross-hatched bars represent CVs derived from 2 studies of physiological variation.[8,9] The white bars represent CVs derived from clinician and laboratorian opinion surveys. If an investigator provided 2 or more CVs for an analyte, the normal range CV was selected. Elion-Gerritzen has 3 CVs for each test, the allowable CV at the lower action limit, the allowable CV at the upper action limit and the allowable CV for serial determinations.[4] The symbol "0" for either lower limit or upper limit denotes that no analytical error is allowed. The black bars represent the average monthly CVs of 2 highly precise instruments, the Dupont aca (EI duPont, Wilmington, Delaware) and Kodak Ektachem 700 (Eastman Kodak, Rochester, New York). The right-hatched bars represent estimates of the between-method bias derived from 1976 and 1985 CAP proficiency surveys (BIAS '85 and BIAS '76 respectively).

(Reproduced with permission from Cembrowski GS. Analytical requirements for clinical chemistry. In: Quality assurance in physician office, bedside and home testing. Howanitz PJ, ed, College of American Pathologists, Skokie, Il, 1986. pp 146-163.)

KEY TO INVESTIGATORS: A = Cotlove '70, B = Young '71, C = Tonks '63, D = Barnett '68, E = Campbell '69, F = Gilbert '75, G = Skendzel '78, H = Barret '79, I = Elion-Gerritzen (Lower Action Limit) '80, J = Elion-Gerritzen (Upper Action Limit) '80, K = Elion-Gerritzen (Serial Determinations) '80, L = Skendzel '85, M = Aca '85, N = Ektachem '85, O = BIAS '85, P = BIAS '76.

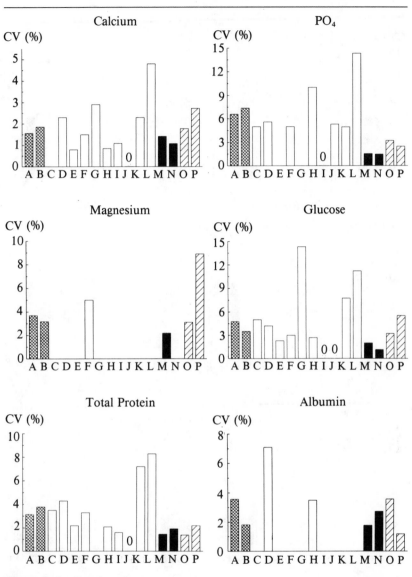

Figure 5–2   Continued.

KEY TO INVESTIGATORS: A = Cotlove '70, B = Young '71, C = Tonks '63, D = Barnett '68, E = Campbell '69, F = Gilbert '75, G = Skendzel '78, H = Barret '79, I = Elion-Gerritzen (Lower Action Limit) '80, J = Elion-Gerritzen (Upper Action Limit) '80, K = Elion-Gerritzen (Serial Determinations) '80, L = Skendzel '85, M = Aca '85, N = Ektachem '85, O = BIAS '85, P = BIAS '76.

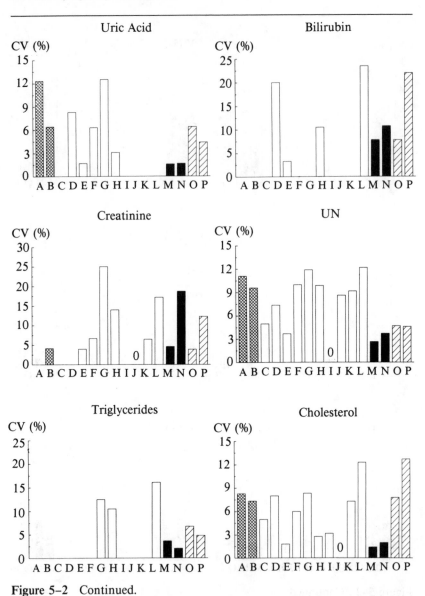

Figure 5–2 Continued.

KEY TO INVESTIGATORS: A = Cotlove '70, B = Young '71, C = Tonks '63, D = Barnett '68, E = Campbell '69, F = Gilbert '75, G = Skendzel '78, H = Barret '79, I = Elion-Gerritzen (Lower Action Limit) '80, J = Elion-Gerritzen (Upper Action Limit) '80, K = Elion-Gerritzen (Serial Determinations) '80, L = Skendzel '85, M = Aca '85, N = Ektachem '85, O = BIAS '85, P = BIAS '76.

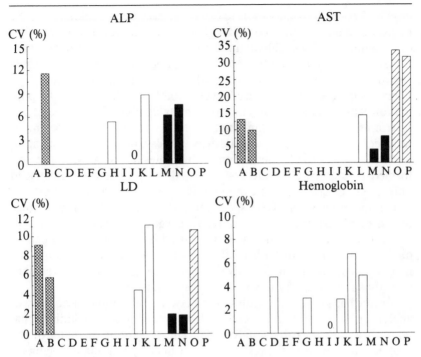

Figure 5–2 Continued.

KEY TO INVESTIGATORS: A = Cotlove '70, B = Young '71, C = Tonks '63, D = Barnett '68, E = Campbell '69, F = Gilbert '75, G = Skendzel '78, H = Barret '79, I = Elion-Gerritzen (Lower Action Limit) '80, J = Elion-Gerritzen (Upper Action Limit) '80, K = Elion-Gerritzen (Serial Determinations) '80, L = Skendzel '85, M = Aca '85, N = Ektachem '85, O = BIAS '85, P = BIAS '76.

and within an individual (intraindividual variation). The measurement of an analyte which exhibits large interindividual or intraindividual variation does not need to be as precise as the measurement of one with small interindividual or intraindividual variation. Cotlove[8] has suggested that the intraindividual and interindividual coefficients of variation ($CV_{Intraindividual}$ and $CV_{Interindividual}$ respectively) could be used to calculate an optimal analytical coefficient of variation (CV_a):

$$CV_a = 0.5 \times [(CV_{Intraindividual})^2 + (CV_{Interindividual})^2]^{1/2}.$$

If 1 coefficient of variation is more than twice the other component, the optimal CV_a is set equal to one half of the larger component.

The 2 coefficients of variation can be determined by taking multiple measurements of a group of individuals and then performing analysis of variance (ANOVA) calculations. Cotlove conducted 2 studies which measured the interindividual and intraindividual variation of multiple chemistry analytes. In the first study, 15 serum constituents of 68 normal subjects were measured weekly for 10 to 12 weeks.[8] The population was diverse, consisting of 35 females and 33 males, and approximately 66% Caucasian. In the second study, blood specimens were collected from 9 young healthy Caucasian male physicians at weekly intervals for 10 weeks.[9] In both studies, the analyses were performed in duplicate. In the first study, the specimens were analyzed on the day of collection; in the second, the serum samples were collected and frozen; all of the specimens were analyzed within a single day to minimize the effects of analytical variation. The optimal analytical CV_a from both studies are presented in Figure 5–2, and can be distinguished from the other estimates by their cross-hatching. The magnitude of the physiologically derived CVs is generally in agreement with those obtained by physician surveys and interviews.

Fraser has studied the within and between individual variability of analyte concentration in patients with diverse illnesses, including renal failure[10] and myocardial infarction.[11] The variations of many of the analytes are similar to the variations in healthy ambulatory subjects and validates the limits derived by Cotlove. Fraser has also presented analytical goals for therapeutic drug monitoring based on pharmacokinetic theory and biologic variation.[12] He has recommended that analytic goals be based simply on intra-individual variation, with CV_a being less than or equal to $0.5 \times CV_{Intraindividual}$. Towards this cause, Fraser has compiled the intra-individual variation of 78 clinical chemistry analytes in healthy populations and 21 analytes in various disease states.[13] He has proposed analytical goals for hematology assays based on intra-individual variation.[14]

Other Approaches

In a 1963 evaluation of 170 Canadian clinical chemistry laboratories, Tonks proposed allowable error limits for the deviations of assayed values of external proficiency specimens from their target values.[15] Tonks' limits were computed from an empirical formula based on the normal range:

$$\text{Allowable limits (\%)} = \pm \frac{(0.25 \times \text{Normal Range}) \times 100}{\text{Mean of Normal Range}}.$$

For analytes with broad normal ranges resulting in allowable error greater than 10% (eg, glucose, phosphorus, urea nitrogen, and cholesterol) Tonks set the upper limit for allowable error as ±10%. The allowable error limits for the other analytes follow: sodium, ±1.8%; chloride, ±2%; and total protein, ±7%. Traditionally, allowable error limits have been considered as 95% confidence limits and correspond to twice the standard deviation of the analytical method. Tonks' allowable errors thus correspond to twice the CV. The allowable CV is obtained by dividing Tonks' allowable error limits by 2. Tonks' allowable error estimates are compared to other estimates in Figure 5-2.

Other approaches have been used to determine maximum allowable error, including mathematical statistical models which incorporate physiologic variation[16] and cost benefit analysis.[17] These approaches, while having merit, have limited application and are too complex for detailed discussion here. One other approach has been used to determine maximum allowable error: using state of the art analytical performance as an ultimate limit for allowable error. Figure 5-2 shows one such set of allowable errors determined in 1975 by Gilbert.[18] Cholesterol measurement has received much attention because of the relationship of cholesterol and coronary heart disease. The Laboratory Standardization Panel of the National Cholesterol Education Program has recommended, as a national goal, an allowable CV of 3% at a medical decision level concentration of 240 mg/dl.[19]

Figure 5-2 compares the diversity of recommended medically allowable CVs to the CVs of the Kodak Ektachem 700 and the Dupont aca. These CVs will be interpreted differently, depending on the background and motivation of the concerned individual. The unsophisticated clinician may demand no analytical error. The instrument maker, on the other hand, may be reluctant to design instruments with precisions equal to those of state of the art instruments, and may thus opt to accept allowable CVs which correspond to the upper limits illustrated in Figure 5-2. This acceptance of these high CV limits is especially common in the design of instrument and methods for physician office laboratories.

The laboratorian can be placed in an uncomfortable situation, having to choose between good precision and low cost. When selecting an instrument, the laboratorian must carefully evaluate its practicality and reliability characteristics (Table 1-2) but place a premium on precision and accuracy. Estimates of within-instrument precision, both short- and long-term, are available from the manufacturer, who must submit these data to the Food and Drug Administration before an analyzer can be marketed for clinical use. Manufacturer-supplied CVs may be optimal, having been derived under controlled conditions by skilled operators (although most manufacturers actually claim larger CVs actually obtained, to ensure that most users will observe performance that meets the claims when they measure CV in their own laboratories). Realistic estimates can often be obtained from published evaluations and discussions with instrument owners. Indirect evidence of intra-instrument precision is available from external proficiency testing. An instrument which exhibits a high interinstrument standard deviation has calibration or precision problems.

It is intuitively apparent that instruments with low analytical CVs should be selected; however, it is not clear what CV is required for specific quality control procedures to detect errors exceeding medically allowable levels. The next section relates a method's inherent precision to the medically allowable error and the magnitudes of errors which a control system must be able to detect to achieve acceptable error levels.

DERIVATION OF THE CRITICAL ANALYTICAL ERROR

Figure 5–3 shows 2 frequency histograms; the top histogram represents the distribution of results from repetitive testing of a single sample with an analytical process exhibiting only its inherent random error, and the bottom histogram represents the distribution of results observed when additional random error is present. The limits on Figure 5–3 correspond to the maximum clinically allowable error, and are labelled as $\bar{x} \pm E_a$, where E_a represents the maximum clinically allowable error. In the top histogram, none of the results extends beyond these limits, indicating that all of the measurements are clinically acceptable. In the bottom figure, 1% of the results exceed the $\bar{x} \pm E_a$ clinical limits, indicating an analytical process which is producing some clinically unacceptable results.

What proportion of the population tested should we permit to have errors exceeding E_a? An analytical process which is capable of producing 999 clinically acceptable answers and only 1 unacceptable result would be very acceptable for most purposes (error prevalence of 0.1%), whereas one which produces 900 acceptable results and 100 unacceptable results would not be tolerated (error prevalence of 10%). Most laboratorians agree that the error prevalence of an analytical process should not exceed 5% and some believe that the prevalence should not exceed 1%. The question has not been answered definitively; eventual consensus standards for error prevalence will probably depend upon the analyte and the use being made of the results. However, since many

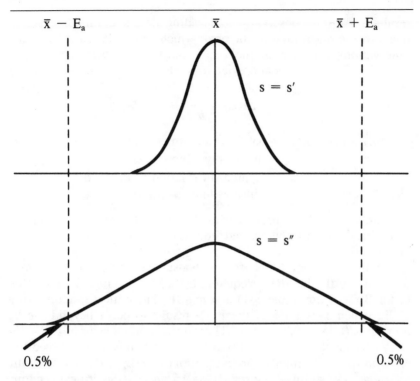

Figure 5–3 Frequency histograms of control data illustrating the derivation of critical random error (ΔRE_c). The inherent random error in the top histogram is $s = s'$. In the bottom histogram, the random error is increased so that the total $s = s''$, which causes 1% of the observations to be outside the $\bar{x} \pm E_a$ limits.

laboratories use a single instrument or method to measure a particular analyte, the most stringent standard will probably apply.

Given the standard deviation of a method, probability theory can be used to derive the limits which result in error prevalences of 1% (or 5%). Referring to Figure 5–3, if an analytical process has an inherent standard deviation, s', then 1% of the results from testing a single sample will be outside the $x \pm 2.58s'$ limits. If $2.58s'$ is less than E_a, the inherent random error of the process is acceptable. For an analytical process yielding 1% of the results outside the $x \pm E_a$ limits, the value of the corresponding standard deviation, s'', would be $s'' = E_a/2.58$. The ratio of s'' to s', given by $E_a/2.58s'$, is the magnitude of random error, expressed in multiples of the usual standard deviation, which

93

results in 1% of the observations exceeding the $\bar{x} \pm E_a$ limits. Westgard refers to the magnitude of the error which causes 1% (or 5%) of the observations to be outside the $\bar{x} \pm E_a$ limits as the *critical* error. The *critical random error* is abbreviated as ΔRE_c, and is obtained from

$$\Delta RE_c = \frac{E_a}{2.58s'},$$

Eq. 5-1

where ΔRE_c = critical random error,
E_a = medically allowable error,
s' = standard deviation of the method during stable operation.

The probability that a particular quality control procedure will detect this critical error can be derived from the appropriate power function plot.

To illustrate, for a BUN assay with a standard deviation of 0.8 mg/dL at 14 mg/dL, the ΔRE_c is equal to $E_a/(2.58 \times 0.8$ mg/dL). Barnett's E_a for BUN (from Table 5-1) is 4 mg/dL. The critical random error ΔRE_c, which causes 1% of the BUN results to occur beyond the E_a limits is $4/(2.58 \times 0.8)$ or 1.9s. Thus, if the random error of the BUN assay is doubled, more than 1% of the observations would exceed the error limits of $\pm$ 4 mg/dL. For a calcium assay ($E_a = 0.5$ mg/dL) with a standard deviation of 0.2 mg/dL at 9.5 mg/dL, the critical random error which results in 1% of the results exceeding $\pm$ E_a limits is $0.5/(2.58 \times 0.2)$, or 1.0s. Even when there is no added random error, approximately 1% of the results are outside the $\pm$ 0.5 mg/dL limits. The situation is worse for a sodium assay ($E_a = 4$ mmol/L), with a standard deviation of 2 mmol/L at 140 mmol/L. The critical random error is $4/(2.58 \times 2)$ or 0.8s. More than 1% of the results are already outside the $\pm$ 4 mmol/L limits.

For many analytes analyzed on common chemistry analyzers an error prevalence of 1% is unachievable. For this reason, a 5% prevalence of errors exceeding E_a is frequently accepted as a performance standard. When there is no added error, 5% of results will exceed $\pm$ 1.96s' limits. The critical random error which corresponds to the 5% error prevalence is thus

$$\Delta RE_c = \frac{E_a}{1.96s'}$$

Eq. 5-2

When 5% error limits are used, the critical random errors for the preceding examples are increased: BUN, 2.6s (5% limits) v 1.9s (1%

limits); calcium, 1.3s (5% limits) v 1.0s (1% limits); and sodium, 1.0s (5% limits) v 0.8s (1% limits). Quality control procedures have more opportunity to detect the increased error before its prevalence exceeds 5%.

The *critical systematic error*, ΔSE_c, is the magnitude of shift which causes 1% (or 5%) of the results to exceed one of the $x \pm E_a$ limits. Figure 5–4 illustrates the results of repeated testing of the same sample with 2 analytical processes, one exhibiting its inherent random error (standard deviation = s') and the other exhibiting the same inherent error plus a systematic shift of ΔSE. If a maximum error prevalence of 1% is being considered, then the distance from the new mean to the point of the distribution representing the outer 1% of the results is 2.33s'. From Figure 5–4, the clinically allowable error is thus equal to the critical systematic error plus 2.33 s', or

$$E_a = \Delta SE_c + 2.33s', \qquad \text{Eq. 5–3}$$

or

$$\Delta SE_c = E_a - 2.33s'. \qquad \text{Eq. 5–4}$$

For a maximum error prevalence of 1%, the critical systematic errors for the BUN, calcium, and sodium analyses referred to above are 2.5 mg/dL, 0.0 mg/dL, and -0.8 mmol/L. Only a small shift is allowed in BUN and no shift is permitted in calcium. The negative value for ΔSE_c for sodium indicates that too much random error is already present in the analytical process. Maximum error prevalences of 1% are unachievable for many analytes.

The magnitudes of the above values of ΔSE_c were expressed in concentration units. It is preferable to have these systematic errors expressed in multiples of the standard deviation, s', in order to evaluate the required P_{ed} from power functions. The critical systematic error may be expressed in multiples of the standard deviation by dividing Equation 5–4 by s':

$$\Delta SE_c = \frac{E_a}{s'} - 2.33. \qquad \text{Eq. 5–5}$$

If a maximum error prevalence of 5% is being considered, then the critical systematic error, expressed in multiples of the standard deviation is

$$\Delta SE_c = \frac{E_a}{s'} - 1.65. \qquad \text{Eq. 5–6}$$

95

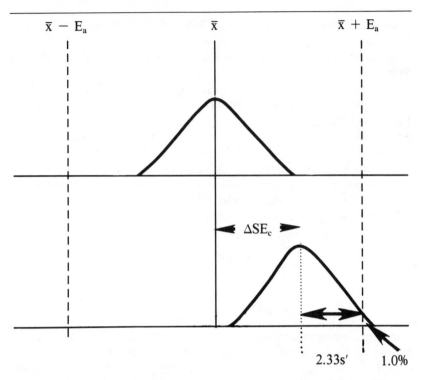

Figure 5-4 Frequency histograms of control data illustrating the derivation of critical systematic error (ΔSE_c). The inherent random error in the top histogram is $s = s'$. In the bottom histogram, the mean is shifted by ΔSE_c causing 1% of the observations to be outside the $\bar{x} + E_a$ limit.

The distance from the new mean to the point representing the outer 5% of the observations is 1.65s'. The critical systematic errors, expressed as multiples of the systematic error, for a maximum error prevalence of 5% are 3.4s for BUN, 0.8s for calcium, and 0.4s for sodium. Use of the 5% error limits indicates that relatively small shifts are clinically allowable for calcium and sodium, and a large shift is allowable for BUN.

Table 5-2 compares the critical random and systematic errors (5% error limits) for selected chemistry analytes for the 2 representative automated chemistry analyzers used as examples in Table 5-1. Virtually every automated chemistry analyzer has one or more methods for which its performance falls short of medically required performance, even when the performance standard is stated as a 95% limit of

96

Table 5–2 Calculation of critical random and systematic errors.

Analyte	E_a	standard deviation aca	standard deviation 700	ΔRE_c, s aca	ΔRE_c, s 700	ΔSE_c, s aca	ΔSE_c, s 700
Albumin, g/dL	0.50	0.06	0.09	4.25	2.83	6.68	3.90
Bilirubin, mg/dL	0.40	0.08	0.11	2.55	1.85	3.35	1.99
Calcium, mg/dL	0.50	0.12	0.20	2.13	1.28	2.52	0.85
Chloride, mmol/L	4.0	1.43	1.21	1.43	1.69	1.15	1.66
Cholesterol, mg/dL	14.4	3.36	4.80	2.18	1.53	2.63	1.35
CO_2, mmol/L	2.0	1.14	1.38	0.90	0.74	0.10	−0.20
Glucose, mg/dL	10.0	2.00	1.20	2.56	4.25	3.35	6.68
Phosphorous, mg/dL	0.50	0.13	0.10	1.96	2.55	2.20	3.35
Potassium, mmol/L	0.50	0.07	0.09	3.64	2.83	5.49	3.91
Sodium, mmol/L	4.0	1.35	1.65	1.51	1.23	1.31	0.77
Protein, g/dL	0.60	0.10	0.13	3.06	2.35	4.35	2.97
BUN, mg/dL	4.0	0.73	1.00	2.80	2.04	3.83	2.35
Uric acid, mg/dL	1.0	0.10	0.10	5.10	5.10	8.35	8.35

Abbreviations: ΔRE_c = critical random errors. ΔSE_c = critical systematic error.

Note: ΔRE_c and ΔSE_c result in 5% of the results exceeding medically allowable error limits (E_a) for the Dupont aca and the Ektachem 700. E_a was derived from Barnett's recommended medically allowable error limits (see Table 5–1). Standard deviations are at medical decision level concentrations from Table 5–1. Any value of ΔRE_c less than 1s or ΔSE_c less than 0 indicates that, even with no additional error, more than 5% of the results already exceed E_a.

error. Given the relatively weak error detection of most common quality control procedures when ΔRE_c and ΔSE_c are less than 2, the analytic errors of many present methods cannot be controlled effectively within 95% limits of allowable error.

Recall that these limits of medically allowable error include all errors of the testing process, not just the analytic errors. If the analytical method takes up all of the error allowance, no error is permitted in the rest of the testing process.

Westgard and Barry have set the criterion for judging the acceptability of a method's stable performance at a 1% limit of error,[20] ie, when the method has only its inherent error, no more than 1% of the data can exceed the ± E_a limits. Control procedures can then be selected so that no more than 5% of the data are outside these limits. The difference between the 1% tolerance for judging inherent error against medically allowable error and the 5% tolerance for allowable error is the zone in which the quality control system operates. This zone is the area into which the method's performance can deteriorate before the analytical errors exceed allowable error on more than 5% of the samples.[21]

Clearly, for many analytes, the inherent performance of many automated analyzers is not acceptable according to published standards. The laboratory community needs to reexamine the standards for these analytes; substandard performance is currently being accepted; is it really medically unsatisfactory? If these performance standards cannot be relaxed, then more precise methods must be developed for these analytes. Otherwise, they cannot be controlled within the required error limits with reasonable quality control procedures.

REFERENCES

1. Barnett RN: Medical significance of laboratory results. Am J Clin Pathol 50:671-676, 1968.

2. Skendzel LP: How physicians use laboratory tests. JAMA 239:1077-1080, 1978.

3. Skendzel LP, Barnett RN, Platt R: Medically useful criteria for analytic performance of laboratory tests. Am J Clin Pathol 83:200-205, 1985.

4. Elion-Gerritzen WE: Analytic precision in clinical chemistry and medical decisions. Am J Clin Pathol 73:183-195, 1980.

5. Campbell DG, Owen JG: The physician's view of laboratory performance. Aust Ann Med 18:4-6, 1969.

6. Barrett AE, Cameron SJ, Fraser CG, Penberthy LA, Shand KL: A clinical view of analytical goals in clinical biochemistry. J Clin Pathol 32:893-896, 1979.

7. Shephard MDS, Penberthy LA, Fraser CG: Analytical goals for quantitative urine analysis: a clinical view. Clin Chem 27:1939-1940, 1981.

8. Cotlove E, Harris EK, Williams GZ: Biological and analytic components of variation in long-term studies of serum constituents in normal subjects. III. Physiological and medical implications. Clin Chem 16:1028-1032, 1970.

9. Young DS, Harris EK, Cotlove E: Biological and analytic components of variation in long-term studies of serum constituents in normal subjects. IV. Results of a study designed to eliminate long-term analytic deviations. Clin Chem 17:403-410, 1971.

10. Fraser CG, Williams P: Short term biological variation of plasma analytes in renal disease. 29:508-510, 1983.

11. Fraser CG, Hearne CR: Components of variance of some plasma constituents in patients with myocardial infarction. Ann Clin Biochem 29:553-557, 1982.

12. Fraser CG: Desirable standards of performance for therapeutic drug monitoring. Clin Chem 33:387-389, 1987.

13. Fraser CG: The application of theoretical goals in proficiency testing based on biological variation. Arch Path Lab Med 112:404-409, 1988.

14. Fraser CG: Desirable standards for hematology tests: a proposal. Am J Clin Pathol 88:667-669, 1987.

15. Tonks DB: A study of the accuracy and precision of clinical chemistry determinations in 170 Canadian laboratories. Clin Chem 9:217-223, 1963.

16. Harris EK: Statistical principles underlying analytical goal-setting in clinical chemistry. Am J Clin Pathol 72:374-382, 1979.

17. Groth T, Ljunghall S, de Verdier C-H: Optimal screening for patients with hyperparathyroidism with use of serum calcium observations: A decision theoretical analysis. Scand J Clin Lab Invest 43:699-704, 1983.

18. Gilbert RK: Progress and analytic goals in clinical chemistry. Am J Clin Pathol 63:960-973, 1975.

19. Naito HK, et al: Current status of blood cholesterol measurement in clinical laboratories in the United States: a report from the laboratory standardization panel of the National Cholesterol Education Program. Clin Chem 34:193-201, 1988.

20. Westgard JO, Barry PL: Cost-Effective quality control: managing the quality and productivity of analytical processes. AACC Press, Washington, DC, 1986, pp 44-49.

21. Westgard JO, Barry PL: personal communication, Madison, Wisconsin, 1987.

CHAPTER SIX

Complicating Factors

The performance characteristics of the quality control rules and procedures presented in Chapters 3 and 4 were derived from simulation studies which assumed ideal conditions: that the control data represented exact, unrounded data with a gaussian distribution and without significant between-run variation. Real world laboratory conditions are not ideal; some or all of these assumptions may be violated. Control rule performance may be seriously degraded. Thus, it is important to be able to recognize deviations from ideal conditions, and either minimize their occurrences or implement robust quality control procedures which are less susceptible to their influence.

BETWEEN-RUN COMPONENTS OF VARIATION

The variations that occur between analytical runs may well be the most important reason for a control rule's degradation in performance. For the purposes of discussion, these between-run variations will be divided into long-term and short-term between-run components of variation. Long-term effects are discussed first because their effects are more apparent.

Long-Term Widening Shifts of Control Ranges

Long-term widening of control ranges is usually caused by recalibrations and variations in reagent lots and control materials. Typically, the initial control range of a new lot of control material is derived from the mean and standard deviation of control data accumulated over a preliminary period of 1 month. Control ranges are then checked at monthly intervals and updated. For many modern instrument and reagent systems, the initial 1 month period includes 1 or 2 reagent lots and minimal numbers of calibrations. Fortunately for most methods, the succeeding reagent lots and calibrations result in roughly equivalent control ranges. As more reagent lots are used and further calibrations occur, slight differences in performance occur and cause small shifts in the control observations. The resulting long-term standard deviation, calculated from all of the control observations, will be higher than the preliminary standard deviation, and widens the control range.

There are certain analytical methods which exhibit significant shifts in the control mean following reagent lot changes and recalibrations. As more reagent lots and calibrations are encountered, these shifts in the control mean result in increased long-term standard deviations and control ranges. Four types of long-term shifts can result from reagent lot change, recalibration, or from the control product itself:

1. Shifts caused by recalibration due to inexact matching of calibrations, although performance is stable within each calibration and reagent lot.
2. Shifts caused by change in performance of analytical method, with only specific control materials affected.
3. Shifts caused by change in performance of the analytical method, with both control and patient specimens affected.
4. Drift over time due to control material instability.

Recalibration

Recalibration can result in shifts of both control and patient data. For example, the calibration of 1 popular discrete chemistry analyzer requires the analysis of 2 levels of calibrator in triplicate. While the analysis of each calibrator in triplicate reduces the standard deviation of the mean of each calibrator by a factor of 0.577 $(1/\sqrt{3})$, the standard deviation of each mean is still more than one half of that of an individual test result. Multiple recalibrations, especially on separate days, using separate vials of calibrator, will clearly demonstrate the imprecision of the calibration process. Although use of a third level of calibrator would reduce the uncertainty of the calibration, the imprecision of the calibration cannot be totally eliminated. If recalibration does result in significant shifts in the control data, we recommend further recalibration to re-establish the original performance. Between-calibration variation must be minimized, as it will significantly increase the long-term standard deviations of controls and reduce sensitivity to error.

101

Manufacturers of instrument systems with long-term reagent and calibration stability provide a recalibration schedule for reagents in use, typically 15 days, 30 days, or 90 days after the prior calibration. If the control data within a reagent lot indicate a stable analytical process, scheduled recalibration may not be required, and the variation of the method can be minimized by not recalibrating. Continuing careful observation of the control data for significant analytical error should determine the need for recalibration. Given the general insensitivity of control rules to small systematic errors, more sensitive counting rules, like 4_{1s} and 10_x, are required to quickly detect the need for recalibration.

A more satisfactory alternative for verifying the accuracy of the present calibration is to analyze the calibrators at the intervals recommended by the manufacturer, and check their reported values against the values expected during a recalibration. If the observed differences are excessive, the method should be recalibrated. This verification procedure is increasingly being recommended by manufacturers of instruments with low between-reagent lot variability. Whenever the method is recalibrated, additional controls should be run after the recalibration in order to increase sensitivity to shifts (see Chapter 8).

Change in Performance of Method Affecting Controls

Occasionally, reagent lot changes lead to dramatic shifts in results for certain control materials but not in patient specimen results. These shifts have been observed in immunoassays. These shifts are probably caused by between-lot differences in antibody behavior toward specific control materials. When shifts are encountered and only control materials are affected, control limits should be calculated using the new lot mean and the usual within-lot standard deviation. Control limits should not be widened. The following example was observed in one of our laboratories and demonstrates how widening the control limits to allow for large between-lot variations may dramatically degrade the performance of a control procedure.

An elevated control product for therapeutic drugs was analyzed with one lot of reagents and yielded theophylline results with a mean of 25.83 and standard deviation of 0.81 µg/mL. Testing with a subsequent reagent lot yielded a mean of 28.68 and standard deviation of 1.00 µg/mL. Recalibration did not correct the shift. Patient results did not reflect the shift. Quality control limits could be set from either the new control mean and typical standard deviation (28.68 and 1.00 µg/mL, respectively) or from limits which would pool results from both lots (mean of 27.26 and standard deviation of 1.70 μg/mL). Use of the $1_{3s}/2_{2s}/R_{4s}$ control procedure with two controls per run and limits calculated from the new mean and a typical standard deviation resulted in a P_{ed} of 0.88 for a shift of 3.0 μg/mL. With limits calculated from the pooled standard deviation, the P_{ed} for a shift of 3.0 μg/mL is reduced to 0.31!

When a reagent lot change results in a control shift, a simple experiment will determine whether the patient data are similarly affected. A group of patient specimens should be analyzed with both the old and new reagent lots, and the average difference (bias) of the 2 sets of determinations calculated. The bias is then tested for statistical significance with a t-test. The number of patient specimens which must be analyzed using the old and the new reagent lots depends on the size of the apparent shift. If the apparent shift is 1 standard deviation, and the user wishes to have a 95% probability of detecting the shift in patient specimens with a t-test significant at p = 0.05, 26 patient specimens must be tested. For shifts of 1.5, 2, 2.5, and 3 standard deviations, the numbers of patient specimens to be tested drops to 12, 7, 5, and 3, respectively.[1] In the theophylline example above, only 3 patient specimens would need to be tested because the shift is 3.5 standard deviations. When small shifts are encountered, it may be prudent to assume that patient specimens are affected rather than trying to prove that they are not. Furthermore, small shifts may not be detected in control data until after several runs, and by then the old reagent lot often has been exhausted.

Shifts Caused by Change in Performance of the Analytical Method; Patient and Control Specimens Affected

When recalibration or new reagent lots produce shifts which affect both patient and control results, the impact of the shift on the total error (the sum of the random error and systematic error) must be assessed. In Chapter 5, random error and systematic error were considered separately when we determined critical error levels which resulted in either 1% or 5% of the observations exceeding the medically allowable limits. Unfortunately, random and systematic errors coexist in the real world laboratory, and their sum must be compared to medically allowable analytic error (E_a). If the sum of random and systematic error is less than E_a, then the shift is acceptable. Quality control ranges may then be shifted accordingly with control limits derived from the new mean and the typical within-lot standard deviation. (Use of the within-lot standard deviation will provide optimal sensitivity to errors.) If the sum of random and systematic error exceeds E_a, the magnitude of the shift is unacceptable, and either the shift or the random error must be reduced.

The total error, the sum of the random and systematic error, is calculated from the following formula[2]:

Total error = random error + systematic error,
Total error = ns_t + SE. $\qquad\qquad$ Eq. 6-1

where
$\quad$ n $\;=\;$ 1.96 or 2.58, corresponding to either the 95% or 99% error
$\qquad\qquad$ limits, respectively,
$\quad s_t\;=\;$ long-term standard deviation,
$\quad$ SE = systematic error.

The total error must be less than E_a:
ns_t + SE < E_a. $\qquad\qquad$ Eq. 6-2

Selection of the multiplier, n, which determines the error limits is important. In Chapter 5, E_a was described as a 99% (or 95%) limit of error; the method's analytical error could exceed E_a on no more than 1% (or 5%) of the samples tested. For a stable analytical method without added random or systematic error, Westgard recommends that 99% of the observations should have a total error less than E_a.[3] In the presence of added random or systematic error, the quality control system might be able to detect error before more than 5% of the observations exceed the E_a limits. Random error at the 99% confidence level is equal to $2.58s_t$, where s_t is the long-term standard deviation. Thus, the criterion for judging the acceptability of long-term total error is given by

$$2.58s_t + SE < E_a. \qquad\qquad \text{Eq. 6-3}$$

The systematic error component can be divided into 2 subcomponents, a constant component (SE_{const}) which is methodology-dependent, and a variable component (ΔSE_{var}) which is calibration-dependent. The constant component can be estimated from proficiency surveys by the deviation from the "correct" value averaged over several proficiency test challenges. The constant component can also be estimated from a split-sample comparison to a reference method. Significant constant systematic error is usually not present, and the total error is assumed to be equal to random error, or $2.58s_t$. If the random error is already large without considering the systematic error, steps must be taken to reduce either the random error or systematic error, or both, if at all possible.

If the random error is acceptable, the acceptability of the shift should be considered. Figure 6-1 shows the distribution of control data before and after a shift due to a change in reagents. To assess the medical significance of the shift, consider the proportion of shifted control values which exceed the $\bar{X}_A \pm E_a$ control limits. The shift is unacceptable if more than 1% of observations exceed these limits. With the new reagents, the previous mean, $\bar{X}_A$, has been shifted to $\bar{X}_B$, the mean of the new reagent lot. The variable component of the systematic error, ΔSE_{var}, is simply

$$\Delta SE_{var} = \bar{X}_B - \bar{X}_A. \qquad \text{Eq. 6-4}$$

The total systematic error is equal to the sum of the constant and variable components

$$SE = SE_{const} + \bar{X}_B - \bar{X}_A. \qquad \text{Eq. 6-5}$$

The total systematic error is then added to the random error component to obtain the total error (Equation 6-3) and compared with E_a. If total error exceeds E_a, the size of the shift should be reduced if possible.

If total error is acceptable, quality control limits should be calculated using the new mean and a typical within-lot standard deviation in order to maintain sensitivity to error.

The above approach to determining the acceptability of a shift assumes that shifts in the control mean have not already increased s_t excessively; total error may be overestimated. However, the authors prefer to overestimate total error rather than to underestimate it. A treatment which is statistically more rigorous, but considerably more complicated, could be developed from the total error criterion of Midgeley.[4]

Drift Due to Control Material Instability

Control material instability can be indicated by a consistent drift in the monthly control mean independent of reagent changes. This instability can be verified by demonstrating the stability of the method (via proficiency testing or method comparison experiments) *and* the stability of an independent calibrator or control material. The long term standard deviation, s_t, will increase steadily for an unstable control material, and the ability of the control procedure to detect errors will diminish as the control limits are widened. If the drift is caused

$$\bar{X}_a - E_a \qquad\qquad\qquad\qquad\qquad \bar{X}_a + E_a$$

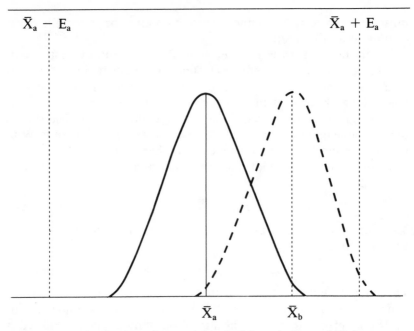

$$\bar{X}_a \qquad\qquad \bar{X}_b$$

Figure 6–1 Distribution of control data before and after a shift due to change in reagents. $\bar{X}_a$ = previous mean, $\bar{X}_b$ = mean of new reagent lot, E_a = allowable analytic error.

by control material instability, limits for control rules should be calculated from an estimated mean and typical monthly standard deviation. If the drift is not too severe, the estimated mean may be calculated as the mean of the last 2 or 3 months' control data. Rarely, the user may need to resort to forecasting the mean for next month by linear regression of the means v time, or by more complex forecasting methods. Procurement of stable control material is the optimal solution. If only a few tests are affected, and the control material will soon be replaced, continual re-estimation of the mean may be indicated.

Short-Term Between-Run Components of Variation

Large control shifts associated with calibration or reagent changes are usually obvious and have readily apparent causes. Their impact on the performance characteristics of quality control procedures can be clearly demonstrated. Other, less noticeable shifts can occur on a daily basis and contribute to between-run variation. Control charts

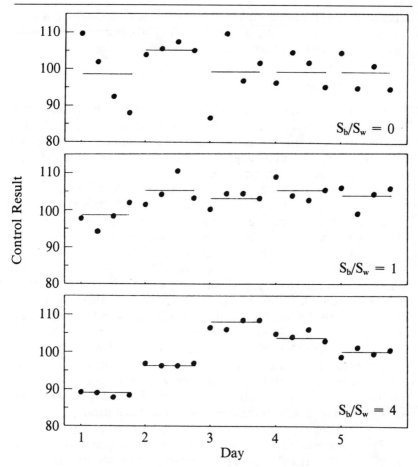

Figure 6–2 Simulated control charts demonstrating the effects of between-run (between-day) variation on the appearance of control data. $\bar{x} = 100$, $s_t = 5.0$. Top: $s_b/s_w = 0$; middle: $s_b/s_w = 1$; bottom: $s_b/s_w = 4$.

illustrating significant short-term (between-day) variation are shown in Figure 6–2, where s_b is the combined between-run and between-day standard deviation, and s_w is the within-run standard deviation. The relationship of the scatter within day to scatter between days is not evident unless the control material is tested several times within each run. When only 1 replicate is analyzed per day, the presence of significant between-run variations may not be evident.

The causes of short-term variation were introduced in Chapter 2.

This section will more completely describe how variation in 4 of these components; control materials, analysts, reagents, and standardization; can result in significant between-run variation.

Control Materials

Some of the variation of an analytical method arises from variability in the control materials used to monitor the method. Since a different vial of control material may be used each day, vial-to-vial differences can result in between-run variation. As mentioned in Chapter 2, these variations are additive as variances.

Control material characteristics which contribute to variation have been reviewed by Ross.[5] Generally, the variation in the filling of the control material vial during manufacture is insignificant compared to the overall variation of the analytical method. The coefficients of variations for the filling of 10 mL vials with lyophilized control ranged from 0.3 to 0.6%;[6] for 5 mL vials, from 0.3 to 0.9%.[7] These vial-to-vial variations can contribute significantly to overall method variation if the method's CV is 1% or less. These vial-to-vial differences can be problematic for the control of sodium, calcium, and chloride. Menson et al reported that large vial-to-vial differences can occur for alkaline phosphatase, acid phosphatase, and creatine phosphokinase.[8]

Reconstitution and subsequent handling of the control material in the laboratory can contribute significantly to between-run variation. The thoroughness of instructions for reconstitution and handling varies widely among manufacturers. The diluent temperature must be standardized for accurate pipetting and stability of certain analytes. Volumetric pipettes must be used for reconstituting lyophilized control materials; unfortunately, less precise serologic pipettes are commonly used in clinical laboratories. Periods of up to 1 to 2 hours may be required for the concentrations of certain analytes to stabilize after reconstitution.[9] For example, alkaline phosphatase activity increases after reconstitution of many control materials. Acid phosphatase activity decreases after reconstitution and must be assayed as soon as possible after reconstitution, unless the control material has been stabilized. Results may be affected by evaporation from the analyzer cup if left uncovered for more than a few minutes. Bacterial contamination in the control material itself or the diluent may dramatically affect stability, especially for controls with claimed stability of several days. Carey et al reported a very high between-run standard deviation for folate method, 4 times the within-run standard deviation,[10] which was later attributed to high bacteria counts in the laboratory water. After sterilization of the laboratory water system, the ratio of the between-run standard deviation to the within-run standard deviation decreased to 1 or less.

Liquid controls, stabilized with high concentrations of ethylene glycol, do not demonstrate the above problems, but exhibit viscosities, osmolalities, and specific gravities which are significantly different from those of patient specimens.[5] They may not behave as authentic patient samples for some analytic methods. Furthermore, they cannot be used on some analyzers because of interactions between the glycol solvent and plastics.

Analyst

Differences in analytical technique contribute to the between-run component of variation. It is important that the same procedure be used by all analysts and be followed as closely as possible. For some procedures there may be as many different variations in technique as there are analysts. This multiplicity in analytical technique can cause large between-analyst variation in technique-dependent procedures, for example, those involving gas chromatographic injections.

Reagents

Reagent preparation and handling may significantly add to between-run variation, even with analyzers utilizing prepackaged reagents. Subtle problems are only noticeable through fairly extensive testing, yet they contribute to s_t. Occasionally, the problems are easier to detect; noticeable variation occurs in the winter when certain isoenzyme reagents freeze during shipment.

Calibration

Between-run variation may be increased by differences in the materials used for calibration and by the calibration method itself. When lyophilized materials are used for calibration, they are subject to all of the concerns described above. Any variation in the lyophilized material is imposed onto the calibration of the method. The calibration curve moves with the calibrator's actual analyte concentration at the time of calibration. If the calibrator's analyte concentration is high because too little diluent was added at reconstitution, then analyte concentrations reported for all samples tested with that calibration will be proportionally low. These problems are most severe when single-vial calibration is used. Use of additional calibrator vials or concentrations diminishes the contribution of calibration to between-run variation.

Between-Run Components of Variation—Simulation Studies

The power functions in Chapters 3 and 4 assumed that all the variation in an analytical method (s_t) occurred within a run. The between-run component of variation, (s_b) representing the between-run and between-day variations, was assumed to be 0. In reality, the magnitude of s_b can be quite large relative to that of s_w, up to 5 times s_w.[10–12] To more conveniently refer to the effects of the between-run and within-run components of variation, we will use the ratio s_b/s_w rather than their absolute magnitudes. Figure 6–2 illustrates simulated control data which contain different amounts of between-run variation (s_b/s_w values of 0, 1, and 4). For the runs with nonzero s_b/s_w the control data cluster around the mean of the run.

The presence of significant between-run variation has 2 effects. First, it increases the long-term standard deviation of the method beyond the inherent within-run standard deviation. The standard deviation is increased from s_w to $\sqrt{(s_b^2 + s_w^2)}$ (see Chapter 2). In effect this causes the sensitivity of the quality control system (the P_{ed} for a given absolute amount of error) to decrease, just because s_t is larger than s_w. Second, significant between-run variation also affects the performance characteristics of the quality control procedures themselves.

Westgard et al have studied the impact of between-run variation with computer simulation procedures.[13,14] For a given control, they assumed that the population of run means was Gaussian and was described by the grand mean of all runs and s_b. In Westgard's simulations, s_b reflects the shorter-term variations described above and not long-term variations which behave more like shifts of the mean. The population of control results within a given run was described by the run mean and s_w. When control data for each run were simulated, the run mean was first generated from the grand mean and s_b, then the individual results within the run were generated from the run mean and s_w.

The simulations presented below represent a wide range of s_b/s_w so that the effects of extreme between-run variations can be demonstrated. For most well-controlled methods, s_b/s_w is generally 1 or less. The reader should become aware of the general effects of increased between-run variations, but should not overinterpret relatively small differences among performance characteristics of different rules caused by between-run variations. The simulation models themselves are not realistic enough for small differences to be significant. Recommendations for some specific situations are summarized in Chapter 8.

Impact on Single-Observation Rules

Figures 6–3A and 6–3B demonstrate how between-run components of variation can affect the detection of random error with the 1_{3s} control rule and 2 controls per run. Control limits for both plots were calculated using s_t, where $s_t = \sqrt{(s_w^2 + s_b^2)}$. In Figure 6–3A, the x axis is expressed in multiples of s_w. Figure 6–3A shows that if errors are considered in terms of s_w, then the presence of between-run variation ($s_b/s_w = 1$ or $s_b/s_w = 4$) reduces the detection of random error present within the run. A very large increase in within-run variation is required (in terms of s_w) to cause control results to exceed the mean $\pm 3s_t$ control limits. With 2 controls per run and an s_b/s_w of 1, s_w must increase to 4 times its original value in order for the increase in random error to be detected 50% of the time. For s_b/s_w of 4, s_w must be very large for the increase in random error to be detected 50% of the time, approximately 12 times its original value. If the control limits are determined from only s_w (mean $\pm 3s_w$) then the P_{fr} increases dramatically in the presence of between-run variation and results in unacceptable performance.[14] If s_t is used to calculate the control limits, as shown in Figure 6–3, the P_{fr} is not increased by increases of s_b/s_w.

Figure 6–3B, power function curves for the 1_{3s} rule with 2 controls per run, considers increased random error in terms of the total standard deviation. Performance *appears* to be relatively unaffected by increases in s_b; however, when $s_b/s_w = 4$, an increase in random error to twice the original s_t represents an increase to twice $\sqrt{[s_w^2 + (4s_w)^2]}$ or more than 8 times the original s_w. Consideration of the performance of quality control rules in terms of s_t does seem to represent reality because the acceptability of a method's inherent random error is usually judged in terms of s_t, and control limits are usually set up in terms of s_t. The random error detection capabilities of the 1_{2s} and $1_{2.5s}$ rules are similarly affected.

Figure 6–4 shows power function curves for the detection of systematic error with the 1_{3s} rule and 2 controls per run. Systematic error is considered only in terms of s_t with the x axis expressed in multiples of s_t. As s_b/s_w increases from 0 to 4, the P_{ed} is reduced by as much as 15% to 20%. The error-detection capabilities of the 1_{2s} and $1_{2.5s}$ rules are similarly affected by between-run variation when 2 or more controls are analyzed per run.[14,15]

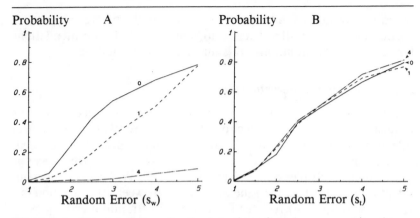

Figure 6–3 Power functions for the detection of random error using the 1_{3s} control rule with 2 controls per run as s_b/s_w varies from 0 to 4. Control limits calculated using s_t. Figure 6–3A; random error axis expressed in s_w. Figure 6–3B; random error axis expressed in s_t. Random error is increased by increasing s_w.

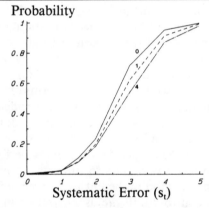

Figure 6–4 Power functions for the detection of systematic error using the 1_{3s} control rule with 2 controls per run as s_b/s_w varies from 0 to 4. Control limits calculated using s_t.

Impact on Counting Rules

In some cases, between-run components of variation may increase the detection of systematic error by some counting rules without in-

112

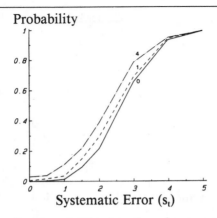

Probability

Systematic Error (s_t)

Figure 6–5 Power functions for the detection of systematic error using the 2_{2s} control rule with 2 controls per run as s_b/s_w varies from 0 to 4. Control limits calculated using s_t.

creasing the P_{fr} to an unacceptable level. Figure 6–5 shows power function curves for the 2_{2s} control rule with 2 controls per run. For a shift of $2s_t$, the P_{ed} increases from 0.22 at $s_b/s_w = 0$ to 0.39 at $s_b/s_w = 4$, while the P_{fr} increases from 0.00 to 0.03. The 4_{1s} rule behaves similarly for 2 controls per run. However, for 4 controls per run, the P_{fr} is 0.04 and 0.15 for s_b/s_w of 1 and 4, respectively. The $8_{\bar{x}}$ rule also behaves similarly for 2 controls per run, and has an unacceptable P_{fr}, 0.15, for $s_b = 1$ and 8 controls per run.

Impact on Multirule Procedures

Figure 6–6 shows power functions for the detection of random error by the $1_{3s}/2_{2s}/R_{4s}$ control procedure with 2 controls per run. In Figure 6–6A, control limits are calculated with s_t for the 1_{3s} and 2_{2s} control rules, and with s_w for the R_{4s} rule. In Figure 6–6B, s_t is used to determine all control limits. Figure 6–6 shows that the probability of detecting random error is much higher when the R_{4s} rule is applied with s_w limits rather than with s_t control limits. With $s_b/s_w = 1$, the P_{ed} for an increase in random error of $2s_t$ is 0.39 using s_w limits v 0.28 using s_t limits. Whenever the same control is run in duplicate (instead of 2 levels of control run singly), the R_{4s} rule can be used with s_w limits to take advantage of this added error detection.

One of the main advantages of multirule procedures is that they allow rules to be applied across controls. To gain this advantage and

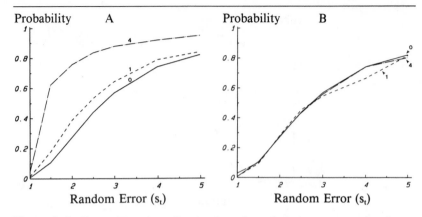

Figure 6–6 Power Functions for the detection of random error using the $1_{3s}/2_{2s}/R_{4s}$ control procedure with 2 controls per run, as s_b/s_w varies from 0 to 4. Figure 6–6A; control limits for 1_{3s} and 2_{2s} rules calculated using s_t; limits for R_{4s} rule calculated using s_w. Figure 6–6B; all control limits calculated using s_t.

maintain an acceptable P_{fr}, s_t limits must be used for all 3 rules. Figure 6–6B shows that the multirule procedure's performance for random error in terms of s_t is not degraded by between-run variation, even when s_t limits are used for all 3 rules. There is a slight increase in the P_{fr} as s_b increases, but the P_{fr} remains at or below 0.04 when there are 2 controls per run.

Figure 6–7 shows power function curves for the detection of systematic error with the $1_{3s}/2_{2s}/R_{4s}$ control procedure with 2 controls. The P_{fr} is increased, and the P_{ed} is slightly increased or decreased depending on the position on the curve.

Figure 6–8 shows power function curves for the $1_{3s}/(2$ of $3)_{2s}/R_{4s}$ multirule procedure for 3 controls per run. Control limits are derived from s_t. Figure 6–8A shows the response to random error and Figure 6–8B, the response to systematic error. In this procedure, the R_{4s} rule results in rejection whenever the difference of any 2 of the 3 controls exceeds $4s_t$. Large between-run variations have little effect on the detection of random error, but cause a decreased P_{ed} for systematic error. The P_{ed} for systematic error is still better than that of the $1_{2s}/2_{2s}/R_{4s}$ rule with 2 controls. Use of s_w limits for the R_{4s} rule will improve the detection of random error, similar to the use of the s_w limits for the $1_{3s}/2_{2s}/R_{4s}$ procedure (Figure 6–6A).

114

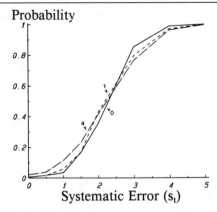

Figure 6–7 Power functions for the detection of systematic error using the $1_{3s}/2_{2s}/R_{4s}$ control procedure with two controls per run as s_b/s_w varies from 0 to 4. Control limits calculated using s_t.

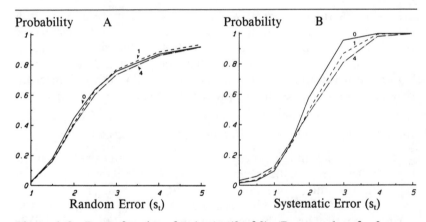

Figure 6–8 Power functions for the $1_{3s}/(2 \text{ of } 3)_{2s}/R_{4s}$ procedure for 3 controls per run as s_b/s_w varies from 0 to 4. Control limits calculated from s_t. Figure 6–8A: random error. Figure 6–8B: systematic error.

Impact on Proportion [(m of n)$_{ks}$] Rules

The effect of between-run variation on the (m of n)$_{ks}$ control rule is dependent on the specific rule and the number of control replicates per run. Figure 6–9 illustrates power functions of the (3 of 8)$_{2s}$ rule for the detection of random error (Figure 6–9A) and systematic error (Fig-

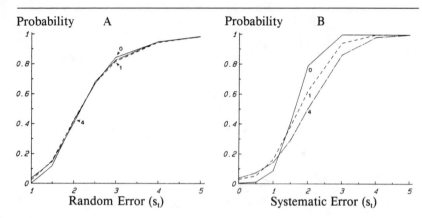

Figure 6–9   Power functions for the $(3 \text{ of } 8)_{2s}$ rule for 8 controls per run as s_b/s_w varies from 0 to 4. Control limits calculated from s_t. Figure 6–9A: random error. Figure 6–9B: systematic error.

ure 6–9B). A run is rejected whenever any 3 or more of 8 controls exceed the mean $\pm$ $2s_t$ limit(s). At least 3 control results must exceed the same control limit, or at least 2 control results exceed 1 mean $\pm$ $2s_t$ limit and 1 control result exceeds the other mean $\pm$ $2s_t$ limit. While between-run variations do not affect the detection of random error, they decrease the detection of shifts whose magnitudes are $1.5s_t$ to $4s_t$.

Impact on Mean and Cusum Rules–Westgard Model

In Chapters 3 and 4, ranges for mean rules were calculated using the standard error of the mean $(s/\sqrt{N})$ as the standard deviation for calculation of limits. For example, the limits for the $\bar{X}_{0.01}$ rule are given by mean $\pm$ $2.58(s/\sqrt{N})$. When either s_w or s_t ($\sqrt{[s_w^2 + s_b^2]}$) is used to derive the control limits, between-run variations lead to a dramatically increased P_{fr}. For a method which is in control, the mean of the controls will have a standard deviation of $\sqrt{(s_b^2 + [s_w^2/N])}$.[16] Using control limits calculated from this combination of s_b and s_w, the decrease in the P_{ed} is dramatic. The power functions in Figure 6–10 demonstrate the effects of between-run variation on the $\bar{X}_{0.01}$ rule and 4 control observations with control limits calculated from s_t and from $\sqrt{[s_b^2 + (s_w^2/N)]}$. These power functions were derived with the Westgard model, in which the run mean was first generated from the grand mean and s_b, then the individual results within the run were generated from the run mean. The Westgard model indicates that between-run

116

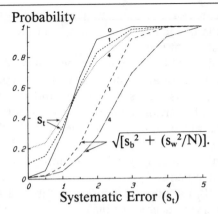

Figure 6–10 Power functions for the detection of systematic error with the $\bar{X}_{0.01}$ rule for 4 controls per run as s_b/s_w varies from 0 to 4. Control limits calculated from s_t and $\sqrt{[s_b{}^2 + (s_w{}^2/N)]}$.

variation has a severe impact on the performance of the mean rule. The effect is pronounced with larger N.

The performance of cumulative sum rules using control limits calculated with s_t is similarly affected by between-run variation;[14] the P_{fr} is dramatically increased.

Douville Model

It is readily apparent from Figure 6–2 that the s_b component represents shifts occurring from one run to another. These shifts have both random and systematic connotations; they can be considered random because they vary from run to run with a standard deviation s_b. However, for a particular run, the shift is really a constant bias (all control samples in a run are affected equally) with the consequence that the mean for the run is shifted compared to the long-term mean (Figure 6–2).

In the Westgard model, systematic errors are simulated by adding a constant value to all control results, thus shifting the overall mean. Varying shifts caused by the between-run component of variation are still present. For a particular run, the bias generated by this last factor can be in the same direction or in the opposite direction as the systematic error. It is therefore possible for a run to have a systematic error (long-term error) offset by the shift induced from s_b. Distinguishing between a long-term systematic error and the effect of the between-

117

run component can be quite difficult. This complication explains the observed reduction of the ability of control rules to detect systematic errors in the presence of significant s_b.

Making such distinctions may not be necessary. When judging the acceptability of a run, we are concerned with the repeatability of the measurements, which is represented by s_w and the bias of that run compared to the stable mean. That bias is equivalent to the difference between the actual mean and the stable mean. In the Westgard model, the average bias of the runs equals the systematic error, but the bias of a particular run is given by the systematic error plus a number generated using s_b. When s_b equals 0, all runs have identical bias. When s_b is not equal to 0, the power functions represent a mixture of runs with somewhat varying degrees of bias.

In order to analyze the control rules' performance as a function of bias (difference between run mean and stable mean), Douville et al proposed an alternate statistical model for studying the effects of s_b.[17] In this model, control limits for the mean rule are calculated from the same combination of s_w and s_b as before. When analytical runs are simulated, performance is evaluated with the same bias for all runs at a particular level of systematic error. When systematic error is introduced, the simulated individual run means are not varied in a distribution described by s_b. Individual results are derived simply from s_w. The term "total shift" is used rather than systematic error to indicate the difference between the run mean and the stable mean. Although the 2 models appear similar, the power functions differ markedly in the presence of significant s_b.

Figure 6–11 demonstrates the Douville model for the performance of the $\bar{X}_{0.01}$ rule with 4 controls per run; these power functions may be compared directly with those of the Westgard model in Figure 6–10 (with limits calculated using the combination of s_b and s_w). With $s_b = 0$, the 2 models provide identical curves because the total bias is equal to the systematic error in the Westgard model. For s_b/s_w between 0 and 1, and with 4 or more controls per run (the usual situation in which the mean rule is applied), power functions derived with the 2 models are very similar. For large s_b, however, the 2 models are quite different, especially for large numbers of controls. With the Douville model, a more abrupt response is seen with a low P_{ed} for shifts below $2.58s_t$, and a very high P_{ed} for shifts exceeding $2.58s_t$. The same phenomenon is observed for the $1_{3s}/2_{2s}/R_{4s}$ combination rule with 2 controls per run in Figure 6–12 and can be contrasted with the Westgard model in Figure 6–7. These abrupt responses reflect the increasing confidence

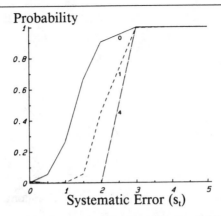

Figure 6–11 Power functions using the Douville model for the detection of systematic error with the $\overline{X}_{0.01}$ rule for four controls per run as s_b/s_w varies from 0 to 4. Control limits calculated from $\sqrt{[s_b^2 + (s_w^2/N)]}$.

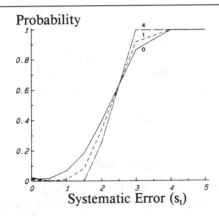

Figure 6–12 Power functions using the Douville model for the detection of systematic error with the $1_{3s}/2_{2s}/R_{4s}$ rule for 2 controls per run as s_b/s_w varies from 0 to 4. Control limits calculated from s_t.

about the amount of bias present; this confidence comes from the relatively low s_w component of random error.

In most situations that the mean rule is applied, where s_b and s_w are of similar magnitude, the 2 models predict similar performance. If s_b is much larger than s_w, the mean rule shows better performance by the Douville model. Regardless, the common message of the 2

119

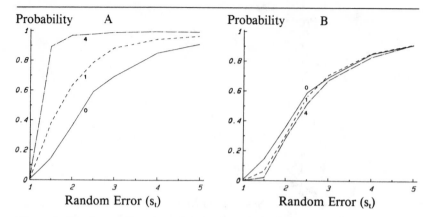

Figure 6–13 Power functions for the detection of random error with the $R_{0.01}$ rule for 4 controls per run as s_b/s_w varies from 0 to 4. Figure 6–13A: Control limits calculated from s_w. Figure 6–13B: Control limits calculated from s_t.

models is that large between-run components of variation are undesirable. Their presence requires that significant control shifts be accepted and obscures the distinction between a daily shift at the limits of acceptability and a new error condition causing an unacceptably large shift.

Impact on Range and Chi-Square Rules

The performance characteristics of the range and chi-square rules for detection of random error are not affected by between-run variation when these rules are applied within-run only, and limits are calculated using s_w. If the x axis of the power function graph is labeled in units of s_t, there appears to be improvement in performance as s_b increases because a small increase in s_t is a large increase in terms of s_w. This effect is demonstrated in Figure 6–13A for the $R_{0.01}$ rule. Actually, performance is still as shown in Chapter 3 (Figures 3–15 and 3–18), when the x axis is labeled in units of s_w.

When limits are calculated using s_t, the P_{ed} and P_{fr} are decreased; however, if the x axis of the power function graph is labeled in units of s_t, there appears to be little effect on performance. The x axis of Figure 6–13B is labeled in units of s_t, demonstrating this effect.

Limitations of Computer Simulation Studies

The effects of between-run variation are not intuitively obvious. Computer simulation procedures are the only effective approach to the study of between-run variation and its effects on the performance characteristics of control rules, but the computer models available for simulation studies cannot take all factors into account.

Neither the Westgard nor the Douville model is entirely accurate. They both treat between-run variations as being normally distributed; however, many analytical methods "wander" within the control ranges and result in non-Gaussian control distributions. Two groups of investigators have reported that the majority of distributions of laboratory data collected over several months were non-Gaussian.[18,19] Visual inspection of their data demonstrated shifts similar to those described in this chapter. If these shifts are not readily detected and corrected, they will result in widened control limits and non-Gaussian distributions of control data. Regardless of the impact of the non-Gaussian distribution, control rule performance will deteriorate simply from the control ranges widening.

Neither the Westgard nor the Douville simulation model allows for between-month variation, which would provide an opportunity to better describe the wandering control phenomenon. To accomplish this task, many months need to be simulated. To simulate 12 months of 4 controls per day and 30 days per month, 1440 data points would be required per simulation; there would be only 12 opportunities for monthly variation to influence the simulations. For simulation studies to demonstrate the effects of monthly variation reliably, there should be at least 300 months of simulations or over 400,000 points simulated!

Rule Selection for Optimal Performance

It is clear that between-run variations distort the distribution of control data; some regions of the distribution are affected more than others. The impact on control rule performance depends on the number of controls per run and whether the control rule uses data from a distorted portion of the population. Thus control rule performance is sometimes subtly affected, and sometimes grossly affected. Table 6–1 presents some generalizations derived from the computer simulations about rule performance in the presence of between-run variation. These generalizations assume that the magnitude of s_b is of the same order as s_w.

Between-run components of variation generally degrade the per-

Table 6–1 Summary of quality control rules and procedures which are affected by between-run variation ($s_b/s_w \geq 1$).

Rules with an unacceptably high P_{fr}
  4_{1s} with $N \geq 4$
  $8_{\bar{x}}$ or $10_{\bar{x}}$ with $N \geq 8$ or 10
  mean rule using s_t limits (Westgard model)
  cumulative sum rules

Rules with the P_{ed} decreased by 15% or more
  single observation rules (1_{2s}, $1_{2.5s}$, 1_{3s} rules)
  $1_{3s}/(2 \text{ of } 3)_{2s}/R_{4s}$
  proportion rules (for systematic error)
  mean rules using combined s_b and s_w limits (Westgard model)
  range rules using s_t limits

Relatively unaffected rules
  $1_{3s}/2_{2s}/R_{4s}$ (slightly increased P_{fr})
  counting rules with low N (slightly increased P_{fr})

Unaffected rule
  Range using s_w limits

Rule with very different performance characteristics
  Mean rule (Douville model)

formance of quality control procedures; thus, they should be eliminated or minimized. Method selection should emphasize avoidance of methods with between-run variation. Between-run variation may be minimized through the following:

1. Rigorous adherence to written procedure. Procedures must clearly state what is to be done in each step in a thorough, easily understood manner.

2. Training of technologists to standardize techniques and procedures and to understand the causes and effects of between-run variation.

3. Selection of calibration materials and procedures which minimize contribution to between-run variance.

4. Selection of control materials with minimum vial-to-vial variation and adherence to specific procedures for reconstitution.

ROUNDING OF DATA

Automated analyzers commonly round results of certain tests to such an extent that analytically significant digits are discarded. Examples of such rounded tests include creatinine (rounded to 0.1 mg/

Frequency

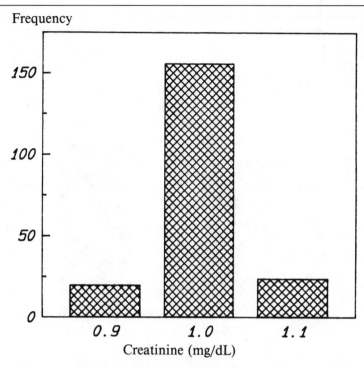

Creatinine (mg/dL)

Figure 6-14 Rounding: histogram of 200 simulated observations from a population with mean of 1.00 and standard deviation of 0.04 after rounding to the nearest 0.1. Control limits calculated from s_t.

dL), bilirubin (0.1 mg/dL), urea nitrogen (1 mg/dL), hemoglobin (0.1g/ dL), and even mean corpuscular volume (1 femtoliter [fL]). The effects of rounding can be observed in tests with a small standard deviation relative to the least significant reported digit. Because the standard deviation is usually proportional to the concentration measured, the effects of rounding are especially noticeable at low to low-normal concentrations where the standard deviations are especially small. The practice of rounding has had the tacit approval of the clinician because the information conveyed by the unreported digit, (eg, the hundredths digit in a creatinine result) lacks clinical significance. Rounding has been further encouraged by some instrument manufacturers and some laboratory information system vendors who are reluctant to produce and handle 2 types of rounded data, one for quality control and the other for patient reporting. The effects of rounding on quality control procedures have been studied by Cembrowski, Westgard, and Groth.[20]

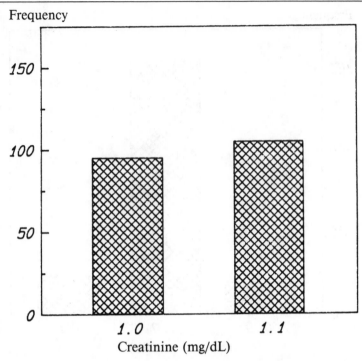

Frequency

Figure 6–15 Rounding: histogram of 200 simulated observations from a population with mean of 1.05 and standard deviation of 0.05 after rounding to the nearest 0.1.

Effects on Calculation of Control Means and Ranges

Creatinine, expressed in mg/dL, may be used as an example to illustrate the effects of rounding. Most automated analyzers can achieve a standard deviation for creatinine of 0.04 mg/dL or less in the normal range, even though the individual results are usually rounded to the nearest 0.1 mg/dL. The frequency histogram representing the creatinine results derived from the multiple analyses of a control material will include very few intervals into which the control data can be grouped. Figure 6–14 represents a simulated histogram of 200 creatinine control results with a mean of 1.0 mg/dL and standard deviation of 0.04 mg/dL. There are approximately 150 observations with a value of 1.0 mg/dL and 25 each of 0.9 and 1.1 mg/dL. The mean ± 1s limits are 0.96–1.04 mg/dL, and they include approximately 75% of the population, v the expected 68%. The mean ± 2s limits are 0.92–1.08 mg/

dL, which round to 0.9–1.1 mg/dL, as do the mean ± 3s limits, 0.88–1.12 mg/dL. The 0.9–1.1 mg/dL range includes all the data. In order for a result to be outside the mean ± 2s or even the mean ± 3s limits, it actually must exceed limits of 0.85 to 1.15. To be outside these limits, the control results must fall more than 3.75s from the mean. The probability of error detection of control rules using the 2s or 3s limits thus will be much lower than those shown in Chapter 3.

Figure 6–15 demonstrates how the location of the mean within an interval affects the distribution of the control data. Simulated data are again presented with the mean shifted to 1.05 mg/dL; the standard deviation has increased from 0.04 to 0.05 mg/dL. The frequencies of observations in the 1.0 and 1.1 mg/dL intervals are almost equal. The mean ± 1s limits are 1.0–1.1 mg/dL, and they represent 100% of the population, v the expected 68%. The mean ± 2s limits are 0.95–1.15 mg/dL, which are usually rounded to 0.9–1.2 mg/dL, and are identical to the mean ± 3s limits, 0.9–1.2 mg/dL. Use of control procedures using mean ± 2s and mean ± 3s limits is likely to be confusing. It is clear from these 2 preceding examples that there will be significant degradation in control procedures using rounded data.

Effects on Control Rule Performance: P_{fr}

The limited number of categories of control observations has a dramatic effect on the performance of quality control rules. If a creatinine assay has a mean of 1.05 mg/dL and a standard deviation of 0.04 mg/dL, the 4_{1s} rule will be severely affected. Consider the probability of false rejection; for the 4_{1s} rule, the P_{fr} should be 0.001 or nearly 0. Before rounding, the mean ± 1s range is 1.01–1.09 mg/dL. Since all results are reported as either 1.0 or 1.1 mg/dL, half the results would exceed the mean + 1s limit and half would be below the mean − 1s limit. The probability that a given result will exceed 1 limit is 1/2 or 0.5. The probability of having 4 consecutive results on 1 side of the mean is $(0.5)^4$ or 0.0625; the probability of having 4 consecutive results beyond either mean ± 1s limit is twice the probability for 1 limit, or 0.125 instead of the expected P_{fr} of 0.001. Computer simulation studies using a mean of 1.05 and standard deviation of 0.04, and based on many runs yielded a P_{fr} of 0.11, in agreement with this intuitive approach.

Figure 6–16 demonstrates how the P_{fr} for the 4_{1s} rule changes as the mean is varied between 1.0 and 1.2 and the standard deviation used to calculate the control limits is fixed at 0.04. The variation of

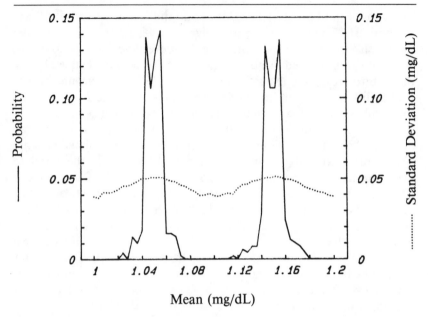

Figure 6-16 Rounding: variation in the P_{fr} of 4_{1s} rule as control mean is varied from 1.0 to 1.2; standard deviation of 0.04 is used to calculate the control limits. The standard deviation of the input observations is not constant but varies between 0.04 and 0.05. Solid line = probability; dotted line = standard deviation.

the P_{fr} is periodic, with a minimum of 0 and a maximum of approximately 0.14. The standard deviation is not constant, but actually varies from 0.04 to 0.05 depending on the mean of the analytical process. The periodicity and the substantial P_{fr} are present for all rules tested. Maximum P_{fr} values and the expected P_{fr} values (without rounding) are summarized in Table 6-2. The 10_x rule had the highest P_{fr}, 0.30.

As the standard deviation increases, the false rejections caused by rounding decrease. Figure 6-17 demonstrates how the P_{fr} is related to the ratio of the standard deviation to the least significant digit (s/LSD). In the creatinine example above, the standard deviation is 0.04 and the least significant digit is 0.1; thus the s/LSD is 0.4. The ratio s/LSD corresponds to number of intervals which are spanned by control observations occupying 1 standard deviation. Because 99% of the control observations will be located between mean−3s and mean + 3s, (range of 6s) the number of intervals occupied by 99% of the observations

Probability of
False Rejection

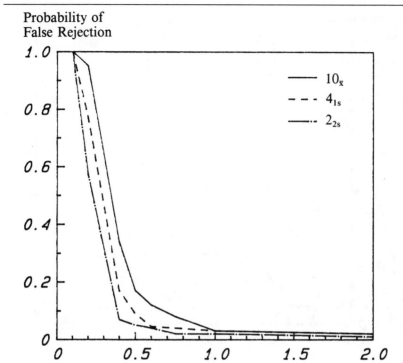

Figure 6–17   Rounding: variation in the P_{fr} of 10_x, 4_{1s} and 2_{2s} control rules with the ratio of standard deviation to least significant digit, s/LSD, varied from 0 to 2.0.

Table 6–2   Effects of rounding on quality control rules.

RULE	N	Expected P_{fr}	Maximum P_{fr}
10_x	10	0.001	0.30
4_{1s}	4	0.001	0.14
$R_{0.01}$	4	0.010	0.13
$(2 \text{ of } 3)_{2s}$	3	0.005	0.12
2_{2s}	2	0.002	0.07
$\overline{X}_{0.01}$	4	0.010	0.06
1_{3s}	1	0.003	0.04

Note: Population mean is varied from 1.0 to 1.2, with control results rounded to nearest 0.1; control limits are calculated using a standard deviation of 0.04.

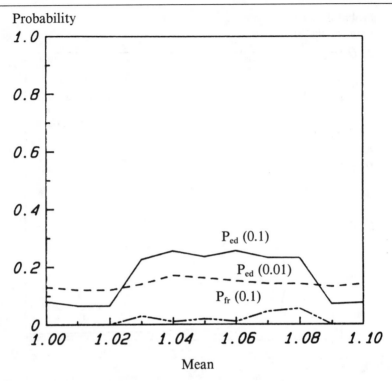

Figure 6–18 Rounding: variation in the P_{ed} of 1_{3s} rule for the detection of a 2s random error as control mean is varied from 1.0 to 1.1. Solid line corresponds to the P_{ed} for data rounded to 0.1; dashed line, data rounded to 0.01. P_{fr} provided for data rounded to 0.1. Standard deviation of 0.04 is used to calculate the control limits.

can be determined from the formula:

Intervals $= 6 \times$ s/LSD.

A s/LSD ratio of 0.4 thus corresponds to 2.4 intervals, roughly 2 to 3 intervals. Figure 6–17 shows that when s/LSD exceeds 1.0, (corresponding to greater than 6 intervals) the P_{fr} is near its minimum value.

Effects of Rounding on Control Rule Performance: P_{ed}

Error detection is also affected by rounding. Consider application of the 1_{3s} rule to the data in Figure 6–14. The mean $\pm$ 3s range is 0.88–1.12 (which rounds to 0.9–1.1). A result must be less than 0.85

Table 6-3 Assays with potential for degradation in quality control rule performance due to rounding. Mean and s_t are for typical control materials on current instruments; least significant digits for patient data are those usually used for reporting patient data, as well as for instrument readout.

Test, Mean	Analytical s_t	LSD for Patient Data
Bilirubin, 1.0 mg/dL	0.025–0.05	0.1
BUN, 15.0 mg/dL	0.4–1.0	1.0
Calcium, 9.5 mg/dL	0.07–0.13	0.1
Creatinine, 1.0 mg/dL	0.04–0.08	0.1
Lithium, 0.6 mmol/L	0.03–0.05	0.1
Magnesium, 2.1 mg/dL	0.08–0.11	0.1
Potassium, 5.0 mmol/L	0.04–0.08	0.1

Abbreviations: LSD = least significant digit.

or greater than 1.15 to exceed 0.9–1.1 limits; thus the actual range in effect is mean $\pm$ 3.5s, the actual rule in effect is the $1_{3.5s}$ rule, and the P_{ed} is decreased from that of the 1_{3s} rule.

The location of the mean within the rounding interval also affects the P_{ed}. Figure 6–18 demonstrates the effects of rounding on the performance of the 1_{3s} rule as the location of the original mean varies in the interval between 1.0 and 1.1. When the control data are rounded to the tenth, the P_{fr} is periodic, with minima at 1.0 and 1.1. When the data are rounded to the tenth, the P_{ed} follows the P_{fr}, with a minimum of 0.06 and a maximum of 0.25. When the control data are rounded to the nearest hundredth, the P_{ed} for doubling of random error is relatively unaffected by the location of the mean. Figure 6–19 demonstrates how rounding causes the 4_{1s} rule to be sensitive to the location of the original mean. Again, when the data are rounded to the tenth, the P_{fr} is periodic, with minima of nearly 0.00 at 1.0 and 1.1, with a maximum of 0.08 at 1.06. The P_{ed} for a shift of 1.5s is approximately 0.30 and fairly independent of the mean when data are rounded to hundredths. When data are rounded to tenths, the P_{ed} tends to follow the P_{fr}, varying from a minimum of 0.00 for a mean of 1.07 to a maximum of 0.83 for a mean of 1.06.

In general, when rounding is severe, the P_{fr} increases and the P_{ed} decreases. Some analytes for which rounding may effect the performance of quality control procedures are listed in Table 6–3. The ratio s/LSD ranges from 0.25 to 1.3; the number of intervals of the corresponding histograms would range from 2 to 10 intervals. Use of an

Probability

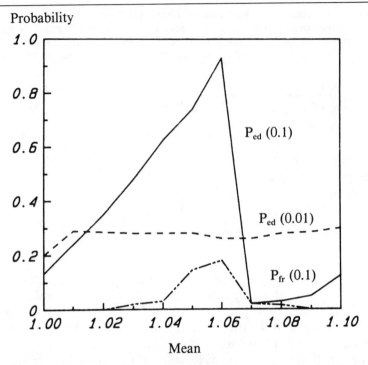

Figure 6–19 Rounding: variation in the P_{ed} of 4_{1s} rule for the detection of a 1.5s shift as control mean is varied from 1.0 to 1.1. Solid line corresponds to the P_{ed} for data rounded to 0.1; dashed line, data rounded to 0.01. P_{fr} provided for data rounded to 0.1. Standard deviation of 0.04 is used to calculate the control limits.

additional digit would increase the number of intervals by a factor of 10, resulting in smoother distributions of control data, and enabling logical combinations of control rules.

When the additional digit cannot be obtained, quality control limits which incorporate rounding must be used. Using the creatinine example again, this time with a mean of 1.0 and s of 0.06, the mean ± 2s limits are 0.88–1.12. If limits of 0.9–1.1 are selected, results outside of the limits 0.95–1.05 will be rejected (mean ± 0.9s limits); if limits of 0.8–1.2 are selected, results exceeding 0.85–1.15 will be rejected (mean ± 2.5s limits). Because of the rounding, no intermediate limits are possible.

In summary, rounding diminishes the amount of information in data; for quality control data, at least 6 different concentration categories are required to prevent serious degradation in the performance of control procedures.

REFERENCES

1. National Committee for Clinical Laboratory Standards: NCCLS proposed guideline EP7-P, interference testing in clinical chemistry. Subcommittee on Interference Testing of the Area Committee on Evaluation Protocols, Villanova, Pennsylvania, 1986.

2. Westgard JO, Carey RN, Wold S: Criteria for judging precision and accuracy in method development and evaluation. Clin Chem 20:825-833, 1974.

3. Westgard JO, Barry PL: Cost effective quality control: managing the quality and productivity of analytical processes. AACC Press, Washington, DC, 1986.

4. Midgeley D: Criterion for judging the acceptability of analytical methods. Anal Chem 49:410-412, 1977.

5. Ross JW: Control materials and calibration standards. In Werner M, ed: CRC handbook of clinical chemistry, vol 1. CRC Press, Boca Raton, Florida, 1982, pp 359-369.

6. Glick JH, Jr: Osmometric estimation of vial-to-vial variation in contents of lyophilized sera. Clin Chem 23:781-782, 1977.

7. Adams TH, Menson RC, Caputo MJ: Comparison of interval variations of Omega with four commercial control sera: implications for improved quality control. Technical Discussion, 43, Hyland Diagnostics, Division of Travenol Laboratories, February 1979. (Cited in Ross, reference 5).

8. Menson RC, Adams TH, Sanford RL: Determination of true vial-to-vial constituent variation by statistical analysis. Clin Chem 23:1120, 1977.

9. Buttner J, Borth R, Boutwell JH, Broughton PMG, Bowyer RC: Provisional recommendation on quality control in clinical chemistry. Part 3. Calibration and control materials, International Federation of Clinical Chemistry. Clin Chem 23:1784-1789, 1977.

10. Carey RN, Tyvoll JL, Plaut DS, et al: Performance characteristics of some statistical quality control rules for radioimmunoassay. J Clin Immunoassay 8:245-252, 1985.

11. Carey RN, Beebe S, Barry PL, Westgard JO: Assessment of performance characteristics of some control rules for retrospective analysis of control data from the IL 508 Chemistry Analyzer. Clin Chem 31:1017, 1985.

12. Aronsson T, Groth T: Nested control procedures for analytical quality control. Theoretical design and practical evaluation. Scand J Clin Lab Invest 44 (suppl 172):51-64, 1984.

13. Groth T, Falk H, Westgard JO: An interactive computer simulation program for the design of statistical control procedures in clinical chemistry. Comput Programs Biomed 13:73-86, 1981.

14. Westgard JO, Falk H, Groth T: Influence of a between-run component of variation, choice of control limits, and shape of error distribution on the performance characteristics of rules for internal quality control. Clin Chem 25:394-400, 1979.

15. Carey RN, Barry PL, Westgard JO: unpublished data, 1987.

16. Westgard JO, Groth T: Design and evaluation of statistical control procedures: applications of a computer "Quality Control Simulator" program. Clin Chem 27:1536-1545, 1979.

17. Douville P, Cembrowski GS, Strauss JF: The influences of the between- and within-run components of variation on the mean rule. J Autom Chem/ J Clin Lab Autom 8:85-88, 1986.

18. Alwan LC, Bissell: Time series monitoring for quality control in clinical chemistry. Clin Chem 34:1396-1406, 1988.

19. Fuentes-Arderiu J, Sierra MT, Pandero AM: No more assumptions about whether control results have a gaussian distribution. Clin Chem 34:769-770, 1988.

20. Cembrowski GS, Westgard JO, Groth T: Effects of data rounding on the performance characteristics of statistical quality control rules. Clin Chem 26:1050, 1980.

CHAPTER SEVEN

Quality Control Procedures Employing Patient Data

LIMITATIONS OF REFERENCE SAMPLE QUALITY CONTROL PROCEDURES

Reference sample quality control is the most widely practiced form of quality control in the clinical laboratory; however, it does not yield perfect error detection. Some of the limitations of reference sample quality control are presented in Table 7–1. Control specimens can detect error conditions only when they are analyzed. The frequency of control analysis has been reduced dramatically as the analytical performance of automated analyzers has become more stable. Only 1 or 2 control specimens are analyzed daily on some chemistry analyzers. The P_{ed} is low when minimal numbers of controls are analyzed; furthermore, no quality control information is provided during the long periods between control specimen testing. Several days may elapse before an intermittent error is detected. Some control is provided by checks of specific instrument function performed by many analyzers; however, only specific operations are monitored. The capabilities of these function checks to detect errors are analyzer-specific and have been formally evaluated on only a few analyzers. Control of overall instrument function can only be achieved by quality control procedures which utilize reference sample or patient specimen results.

The control product can limit the usefulness of the control result. Hematology control products, for example, are expensive and can outdate in as little as 1 or 2 months. The changes of control ranges with each lot change make it tempting for a laboratory to use the manufacturer's recommended control ranges. Use of these control limits reduces the control procedure's sensitivity because these limits are widened by the manufacturer to incorporate interanalyzer variability. The physical properties of the control product may be so different from

Table 7–1 Limitations of reference sample quality control.

May be expensive.

Control materials may be unstable.

Control materials may exhibit characteristics which differ from patient specimens.

Usually monitors analytical stage, ignores preanalytical components.

those of patient specimens that the control product may not reveal an error condition which is affecting the patient results.

Finally, because control specimens are usually introduced to the testing process at the analysis phase (Figure 1–1), controls cannot detect preanalytical factors which can result in error, factors which may be present in the collection, identification, transportation, and preparation phases.

PATIENT RESULTS–FREE QUALITY CONTROL

Patient data can be used to evaluate the testing process, from the ordering phase to the reporting phase. These data can be derived from a single specimen from 1 patient, several specimens from 1 patient, or 1 or more specimens from multiple patients. For some analyzers, the evaluation of patient data may be the first line of quality control when control specimens are not being analyzed. Different control procedures utilizing patient data can detect systematic and/or random error.

Figure 7–1 illustrates how an experienced analyst evaluates new patient data. The analyst first determines whether their values are reasonable. For example, a serum sodium of 20 mmol/L or a serum potassium of 30 mmol/L is impossible and should be followed with inquiries about the type of biological fluid analyzed. The laboratory result may be physiologically possible but so aberrant that it is associated with a life-threatening condition. The analyst must recognize such values and immediately bring them to the attention of the attending physician. Lists of such "panic" or "critical" values are found in all laboratories. Table 7–2 is an adult patient critical value list adapted from the list used at the Hospital of the University of Pennsylvania and the list published by Baer.[1] An approach for reviewing and reporting critical values, developed by Clevenger,[2] is summarized in Table 7–3. Each laboratory must set up a protocol for handling critical values. With increasing emphasis placed on outpatient testing, this protocol should also include how outpatient results will be handled. Alerting

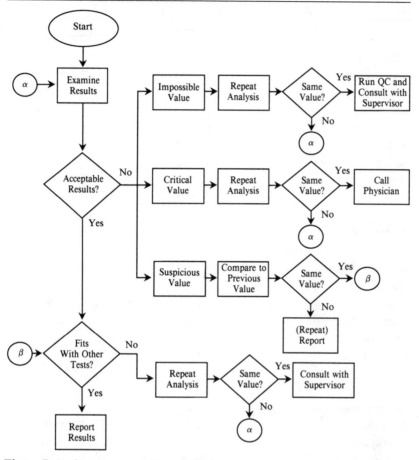

Figure 7–1 Steps employed by skilled technologists in evaluating new laboratory results.

Reproduced with permission. From Cembrowski GS: Use of patient data for quality control. Clin Lab Med 6:715-733, 1986.

the appropriate clinician or the patient can become very involved; on occasion the State Police has been asked to bring a patient to the emergency room when the physician could not be reached and the patient did not have a telephone.

The laboratory result may not be in the life-threatening range but may be sufficiently abnormal to cause the analyst to compare it to the patient's previous result. If the new value is close to the old value, then

Table 7-2 Critical value list for adult patients.

Test	Low Limit	High Limit
Chemistry		
Serum sodium	<115 mmol/L	>160 mmol/L
Serum potassium	<2.5 mmol/L	>6.5 mmol/L
Serum bicarbonate	<10 mmol/L	>40 mmol/L
Serum calcium	<6 mg/dL	>14 mg/dL
Serum phosphate	<1.0 mg/dL	None
Serum magnesium	<1.0 mg/dL	>3.5 mg/dL
Serum glucose	<40 mg/dL	>600 mg/dL
Arterial pCO_2	<20 mm Hg	>70 mm Hg
Arterial pH	<7.2	>7.6
Arterial pO_2	<40 mm Hg	None
Therapeutic Monitoring		
Acetaminophen	None	>150 μg/mL
Amitriptyline	None	>400 ng/mL
Carbamazepine	None	>12 μg/mL
Chloramphenicol	None	>60 μg/mL
Cyclosporine	None	>500 μg/L
Desipramine	None	>400 ng/mL
Digitoxin	None	>35 ng/mL
Digoxin	None	>2.5 ng/mL
Disopyramide	None	>7.0 μg/mL
Doxepin	None	>400 ng/mL
Ethosuximide	None	>200 μg/mL
Gentamycin	None	>12 μg/mL
Imipramine	None	>400 ng/mL
Lidocaine	None	>5.0 μg/mL
Lithium	None	>1.5 mmol/L
Nortriptyline	None	>200 ng/mL
Phenobarbital	None	>50 μg/mL
Phenytoin	None	>30 μg/mL
Primidone	None	>24 μg/mL
Procainamide	None	>12 μg/mL
Quinidine	None	>7.0 μg/mL
Salicylate	None	>30 mg/dL

(Continued)

Table 7–2   Continued.

Test	Low Limit	High Limit
Theophylline	None	>25 μg/mL
Tobramycin	None	>12 μg/mL
Valproic acid	None	>200 μg/mL
Hematology		
Hemoglobin	<7 g/dL	>18 g/dL
Hematocrit	$<20\%$	$>60\%$
White cell count	$<1.0 \times 10^9$/L	$>25 \times 10^9$/L
Platelet count	$<50 \times 10^9$/L	$>800 \times 10^9$/L
Coagulation		
Fibrinogen	<1.0 g/L	None
Prothrombin time	None	>24 seconds
Partial thromboplastin time	None	>100 seconds
Fibrin degradation products	None	>80 mg/L

Modified with permission. From Cembrowski GS: Use of patient data for quality control. Clin Lab Med 6:715-733, 1986. And from Baer DM: Critical values for drug levels. Med Lab Obs 14(8):46-47, 1982.

it is released; otherwise the analysis may be repeated with the new value reported.

The analyst then checks for consistency among the new results. For example, the ratio of a patient's hemoglobin to hematocrit is very constant when determined by multichannel hematology analyzers which use the impedance principle to size and count red blood cells. The ratio, expressed as the mean corpuscular hemoglobin concentration (MCHC), should be approximately 33 g/dL. Significant deviation from 33 indicates either very aberrant red cells or laboratory error in either hemoglobin or hematocrit. Similarly, a markedly increased prothrombin time accompanied by a normal activated partial thromboplastin time is unusual and generally is investigated.

Serum or plasma sodium, chloride, and total carbon dioxide levels are related to one another by the principle of electroneutrality. The charge contribution of the cations (primarily Na^+) should equal that of the contribution of the anions (primarily Cl^- and CO_2^-). The anion gap, usually calculated from the formula $[Na^+] - [Cl^-] - [CO_2^-]$, is a measure of the undetermined anions and should be within 6 to 18 mmol/L for most patients. Deviation outside this range can be due to either electrolyte and acid-base abnormalities or laboratory error. Many

Table 7-3 Protocol for reviewing and reporting critical values.

1. Check the specimen for abnormalities.
2. Check controls to see if they are within range.
3. Rerun controls and specimen(s).
4. Check results on other specimens within run.
5. Check results obtained previously on patient, admitting diagnosis, or current clinical picture.
6. Call nursing station to see if patient is undergoing any special treatment.
7. Redraw the patient, run new patient specimen along with controls (done infrequently).
8. Bring questionable results to attention of the supervisor or pathologist.
9. Call results to appropriate personnel.

Modified with permission. From Clevenger RR. A protocol for verifying critical values. Med Lab Obs 17(5):72–76, 1985.

laboratories investigate specimens with abnormal anion gaps with repeat testing.

Many of the actions of the technologist in evaluating the patient data have been programmed into quality control systems resident in current laboratory information systems (LIS). The LIS can identify patients with analyte values that are beyond critical limits or technical limits (outside of linear range). The LIS can identify patients with large deviations in serial laboratory results. These large changes can be due to therapy, specimen mixup, or instrument error and should be investigated. The LIS can also calculate averages of consecutive patient results generated by a single instrument or operator. A shift in the patient average is consistent with an analytical shift but may also be due to a change in the makeup of the patient population.

This chapter next describes some quality control procedures using patient data, including delta checks, averages of patient data, multivariate checks of patient data, patient replicate checks, and patient sample comparisons.

DELTA CHECKS

If a patient's condition is stable, the patient's serial test results should also be stable. The difference between consecutive test results in a stable patient, referred to as delta (Δ), should thus be small. If a delta is large and exceeds a predefined limit (a delta check failure), it indicates 1 of 3 possibilities: (1) a larger than expected deviation in the measured analyte; the patient's laboratory value really did change, (2) a specimen misidentification or mixup, or (3) an error in 1 of the 2 results used to derive the delta. After Lindberg suggested that large deviations in serial hemoglobin and hematocrit should be investigated,[3] Nosanchuk and Gottmann initiated a 5 year evaluation of a delta check system for hematology.[4] They found that failed delta checks were infrequently caused by technical errors or instrument failures, but more often by real variation in analyte concentration or specimen misidentification. In the hematology laboratory, the variation in serial hemoglobins and in white cell and platelet counts can be extreme, especially with hemorrhage and transfusion. Similarly, clinical chemistry results can change dramatically, eg, electrolyte values with renal dialysis and transplant, intravenous therapy, and potassium supplementation.[5] Since Nosanchuk's paper, the delta check system has been implemented in most LISs with the analyst automatically alerted to delta check failures.

Delta is usually calculated in 1 of 2 ways:

$$\Delta \text{ (test units)} = \text{Result (time 2)} - \text{Result (time 1).} \qquad \text{Eq. 7–1}$$

$$\Delta(\%) = 100 \times \frac{\text{Result (time 2)} - \text{Result (time 1)}}{\text{Result (time 2)}}. \qquad \text{Eq. 7–2}$$

The limits for delta can thus be expressed either in the units of the test or in percentages. Two different approaches have been used to derive delta limits. The more rigorous approach requires the collection of consecutive pairs of patient data representative of the data to be delta checked. The deltas are then calculated and plotted as frequency histograms to determine statistical confidence limits for the deltas, eg, either 95% or 99% limits. Wheeler and Sheiner used such a quantitative approach to determine delta check limits for the directly measured quantities, Na^+, K^+, Cl^-, CO_2^-, creatinine, BUN, and 2 derived parameters, anion gap and the BUN/creatinine ratio.[6] They provided several sets of delta check limits: limits for tests done 1 to 1.5 days apart, limits for tests done 1.5 to 2.5 days apart, and limits dependent on the concentration of the second measurement.

The second approach to the derivation of delta check limits is empirical and requires setting of limits based on intraindividual variation and clinical experience. Because these empirical limits are approximations, their values should be adjusted so they do not identify an excess number of patients as delta failures when they have genuine changes in test values.

Table 7-4 Comparison of delta check limits for routine analytes from 4 references.

Analyte	Whitehurst[25]	Ladenson[26]	Sher[27]	Wheeler and Sheiner[6]
Na^+ (mmol/L)	±6	±5% → ±7	±8	±10
K^+ (mmol/L)	±1.2	±20% → ±0.9	±2	±1.4
Cl^- (mmol/L)	±8		±10	±10
CO_2^- (mmol/L)	±6		±15	±8
Creatinine (mg/dL)	±0.5	±50% → ±0.5	±1	+0.3 to −0.8
BUN (mg/dL)	±5	±50% → ±10	±10	+4 to −18

Note: Wheeler and Sheiner's limits (1–99 percentile limits) were obtained with a quantitative approach; the other limits were derived empirically.

Reproduced with permission. From Cembrowski GS: Use of patient data for quality control. Clin Lab Med 6:715-733, 1986.

Table 7-4 compares the delta check limits used by different investigators for BUN, creatinine, and the commonly measured electrolytes. Because the magnitudes of the quantitatively derived and empirically derived limits are equivalent, approximately the same performance should be achieved by delta check systems using either the empirically or quantitatively defined delta check limits. In fact, when Sheiner, Wheeler, and Moore evaluated 3 delta check systems, they found that when the specificity of the delta check system was fixed at 95% (only 5% of the correctly identified specimens would fail the delta check), the resulting sensitivity of any of the 3 delta check systems was approximately 50% (50% of specimen mixups failed delta check).[7]

At a 1% specimen mixup rate, 5.5% of all the specimens would fail the delta check (5% of the correctly identified specimens plus one half of the incorrectly identified specimens). The predictive value of a failed delta check would thus be 0.5/5.5 or 9%. A very large fraction of the specimens, 91%, would be investigated unnecessarily. Table 7-5 compares the predictive value of a failed delta check for 3 different specificity/sensitivity combinations and various misidentification rates. As the misidentification rate decreases, so does the predictive value.

In the 3 delta check systems evaluated by Sheiner, Wheeler, and Moore, increasing the specificity to 97.5% decreased the sensitivity to 20%.[7] Table 7-5 shows that such an approach does not significantly change the predictive value of a failed delta check.

A novel multivariate delta check approach was employed by Iizaka, Kume, and Kitamura, who computed a delta based on consecutive pairs of zinc sulfate turbidity, cholesterol, and cholinesterase determinations.[8] Because these 3 tests exhibit high interindividual variation

Table 7–5   Predictive value of a failed delta check for correctly recognizing specimen mixups.

Mixup Rate	Specificity/Sensitivity		
	95.0%/50.0%	97.5%/20.0%	98.0%/65.0%
2.0%	16.9	14.0	39.9
1.0%	9.2	7.5	24.7
0.5%	4.7	3.9	14.0
0.1%	1.0	0.8	3.2

and are considered together, the specificity and sensitivity are better than those documented by Sheiner, Wheeler, and Moore,[7] approximately 98% and 65%, respectively. Despite these superior performance characteristics, the predictive value of a failed delta check was very low, approximately 3%, owing to the very low specimen mixup rate, approximately 0.1% (Table 7–5). Such an approach may only be effective in Japan where zinc sulfate turbidity, cholesterol, and cholinesterase are ordered together. In most other countries, an approach which indicates large changes in single analytes is standard.

Delta check systems vary greatly. Table 7–6 contrasts delta check limits which have been programmed into the LISs at the Hospital of the University of Pennsylvania (HUP) and Peninsula General Hospital (PGH). At PGH, different magnitudes of change are allowed, depending on the original concentration of the analyte. Large deviations were permitted at HUP because of limitations in the LIS delta check program. Some laboratorians feel that trends consistent with therapy should not be signaled by delta checks, eg, decreased BUN and creatinine values with dialysis. Such an approach would require an eloquent delta check program but would increase the low predictive value of a failed delta check. Future versions of hospital information systems (HISs) may be able to provide the clinical database to allow advanced, more specific delta checks which would incorporate both clinical and laboratory data.

Whenever a significant delta is detected, it should be systematically investigated; an explanation for failed delta checks usually can be discovered. A sequence for investigating delta failures is shown in Figure 7–2. First, the identification of the specimen in question should be confirmed. Then the patient's cumulative laboratory record and clinical diagnosis should be reviewed. As stated above, most delta check failures represent changes in the patient's condition. For example, uncontrolled diabetes will result in failed glucose delta checks, and its

141

Table 7-6 Comparison of delta check limits for selected clinical chemistry tests used at 2 hospitals.

	HUP	PGH
Acid phosphatase	99%	0–10U/L: 1.5U/L 10–20U/L: 2U/L 20–50U/L: 5U/L 50–200U/L: 10U/L 200–500U/L: 15% >500U/L: 20%
Alanine aminotransferase	99%	0–50U/L: 15U/L 50–200U/L: 30% 200–800U/L: 25% >800U/L: 200U/L
Albumin	50%	0–5g/dL: 0.5 g/dL 5–10g/dL: 0.7 g/dL
Alkaline phosphatase	50%	0–100U/L: 30% 100–200U/L: 50% 200–400U/L: 50% 400–800U/L: 100U/L 800–2000U/L: 200U/L >2000U/L: 300U/L
Ammonia	99%	30%
Amylase	99%	0–50 U/L: 10 U/L 50–200 U/L: 15% 200–1000 U/L: 20% 1000–2000 U/L: 25% 2000–4000 U/L: 300U/L >4000 U/L: 500U/L
Anion gap	99%	
Aspartate aminotransferase	99%	0–50U/L: 15U/L 50–200U/L: 30% 200–800U/L: 25% >800U/L: 200U/L
Bilirubin, total	75%	0–2mg/dL: 0.5mg/dL 2–10 mg/dL: 1.0mg/dL 10–20mg/dL: 2.0mg/dL >20mg/dL: 3.0mg/dL
Bilirubin, direct	50%	0–1mg/dL: 0.3mg/dL 1–5mg/dL: 0.6mg/dL 5–15mg/dL: 20% >15mg/dL: 3.0mg/dL
Bilirubin, Delta (Ektachem)	100%	
Bilirubin, Indirect	75%	0–2 mg/dL: 0.5mg/dL 2–10mg/dL: 1.0mg/dL 10–20mg/dL: 2.0mg/dL >20mg/dL: 3.0mg/dL

(Continued)

Table 7–6   Continued.

	HUP	PGH
Calcium	20%	0–3mg/dL: 0.4 mg/dL 3–8mg/dL: 0.5 mg/dL 8–12mg/dL: 0.7 mg/dL >12mg/dL: 10%
Carbon Dioxide	50%	6 mmol/L
Chloride	20%	6 mmol/L
Cholesterol	50%	0–100mg/dL: 20mg/dL 100–200mg/dL: 30mg/dL 200–400mg/dL: 40mg/dL >400mg/dL: 15%
Creatine Kinase	99%	0–150U/L: 40U/L 150–1000U/L: 20% 1000–4000U/L: 500U/L >4000U/L: 15%
Creatine Kinase—MB fraction	50%	0–30U/L: 5U/L >30U/L: 10U/L
Creatinine	50%	0–2mg/dL: 0.6mg/dL 2–10mg/dL: 1.5 mg/dL >10mg/dL: 30%
Glutamyl Transpeptidase	99%	0–100U/L: 25U/L 100–400U/L: 50U/L 400–1000U/L: 200U/L >1000U/L: 200U/L
Glucose	99%	0–100mg/dL: 25mg/dL 100–200mg/dL: 30mg/dL 200–500mg/dL: 50mg/dL >500mg/dL: 100mg/dL
Glucose, CSF	50%	30%
HDL Cholesterol	99%	30%
Lactate Dehydrogenase (LDH)	99%	0–100U/L: 40U/L 100–500U/L: 75U/L >500U/L: 25%
LDH-1	50%	0–75U/L: 20U/L >75U/L: 30%
Osmolarity	20%	0–300mosm/L: 10mosm/L >300mosm/L: 15mosm/L
Phosphate	99%	1.0mg/dL
Potassium	50%	0–2.5mmol/L: 0.5mmol/L 2.5–5.0mmol/L:0.7mmol/L 5.0–7.0mmol/L: 10% >7.0mmol/L: 0.8mmol/L

(Continued)

Table 7-6 Continued.

	HUP	PGH
Protein, total	30%	0.8g/dL
Protein, CSF	50%	30%
Sodium	50%	10mmol/L
Triglycerides	99%	0-200mg/dL: 40mg/dL 200-600mg/dL: 75mg/dL >600mg/dL: 150mg/dL
Uric acid	50%	2.0mg/dL
Urea nitrogen	75%	0-50mg/dL: 10 mg/dL

Abbreviations: HUP = the Hospital of the University of Pennsylvania. PGH = Peninsula General Hospital.

diagnosis is obvious once the cumulative record is checked. Results failing delta checks should not be accepted simply because other tests on the same specimen demonstrate the same pathophysiological trend; for example, liver enzymes could all show the same trend between the baseline specimen and the suspect specimen, whether a specimen mixup has occurred or not.

The original specimen should be retested if the delta check failure is not readily explained by the clinical diagnosis and the cumulative record. A sample should be taken from the original blood collection tube or urine container in order to detect mixups in aliquoting the specimen.

If the result is confirmed using the original sample, and not explained by the patient's previous data or a change in the patient's condition, a new specimen should be collected and tested. If the new specimen result is different from the original result, the most likely explanation is specimen mixup through phlebotomy error. If any part of the phlebotomy mixup involves Blood Bank specimens, *immediate investigation* is required. Because 2 patients are usually involved, the other patient must be rapidly identified and the mixup's impact on Blood Bank therapy and other laboratory results must be mitigated.

If the result which has failed the delta check is verified by testing the new specimen, the specimen(s) should be retested with an alternate analytical methodology, if available. If no error is discovered, an appropriately worded comment should be placed in the patient record, such as "checked and verified," to inform the clinician that the large delta is real.

A mixup between the original specimen and the aliquot actually tested can arise from 3 different circumstances: (1) mixup of aliquots

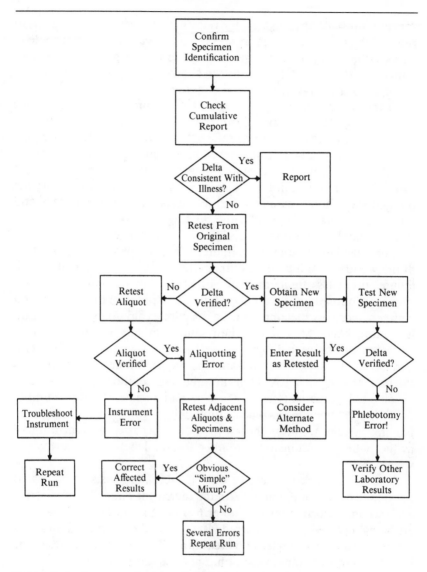

Figure 7–2 Sequence for investigating delta check failure.

of 2 specimens; (2) erroneous aliquotting of the same specimen twice; or (3) an error in the sequence of the patient specimens in a portion of the run. Specimens (aliquots) near the one demonstrated to be er-

145

roneous must be investigated by retesting the original specimens to rule out the mixup of 2 or more specimens. Occasionally, enough delta check failures can occur to make an entire run suspect. If more than 1 mixup is discovered, the entire run should be repeated with samples taken from the original specimen containers.

If the test result causing a delta check failure indicates a serious deviation or exceeds a critical limit (Table 7–2), and the first steps of delta check verification do not refute the result, the patient's nursing staff should be notified of the preliminary result. They should be told that the result is being verified and that they might observe the patient carefully until verification is complete. This practice of notifying the nursing staff should extend to critical tests such as electrolytes and therapeutic drugs. Frequently, the nursing staff will observe changes in the patient's condition consistent with the test result in question.

For most laboratories, outpatient testing comprises a large portion of the workload. While most outpatients are healthy, and delta check failures occur less frequently for outpatients than for inpatients, followup on outpatient delta check failures is problematic. The period between successive testings can be very long; physiological variation is a more likely explanation than sample mixup. Obtaining a new specimen can be very difficult as well as inconvenient to the patient. Discussing the aberrant result and the required followup action with the patient's physician is often the preferred solution. In many institutions, the outpatient receives a new patient identification number for each outpatient "occurrence"; thus, delta failures are not detectable. For this reason, we have chosen the Social Security account number as the patient identification number for the laboratory information system.

The delta check is effective only if laboratory tests are repeated during the course of therapy. With the increasing emphasis on discrete analysis and selective testing, fewer test panels and fewer single tests are being repeated. The reordered tests will be those required for monitoring, such as electrolytes and creatinine. Because most of these tests have low interindividual variation, their usefulness for demonstrating specimen interchanges will be limited. Despite this limitation and the low predictive value of a failed delta check, Wheeler and Sheiner advocate the use of delta check systems.[5] Delta checks can detect preanalytical, analytical, and postanalytical errors; appropriate followup can increase clinicians' confidence in the laboratory and decrease their ordering of unnecessary confirmatory tests.

USE OF AVERAGES OF PATIENT DATA FOR
QUALITY CONTROL

In 1965 Hoffmann and Waid described the use of averages of patient data (also known as the average of normals) for the quality control of chemistry analyses.[9] While many of the subsequent evaluations of Hoffmann's average of patients quality control procedure demonstrated poor error detection capabilities, its use is widespread. Some large chemistry analyzers are able to calculate the averages of patient data selected by test result, truncation limits, and period of interest. Daily patient means are used by some reference laboratories for the detection of analytical drift. Most automated multichannel hematology analyzers use the average of patient red cell indices computed by "Bull's algorithm" to detect systematic error.

Until recently, the error detection capabilities of quality control procedures using the means of patient data were poorly understood. Cembrowski, Westgard, et al, used computer simulations to derive power functions for several quality control procedures which used patient data averages.[10-12] These power functions indicate that averages of patient data can be quite powerful but must be optimized to provide sensitive and specific error detection capabilities.

Average of Patients (AOP)

Hoffmann included patient data for averaging if they were within a reference range previously determined from patient data. The averages were then evaluated with the mean rule using 95% confidence limits for the stable patient mean ($\bar{x} \pm 1.96\ s_p/\sqrt{N_p}$) where s_p was the standard deviation of the patient population and N_p was the number of patients averaged. An error was signaled whenever several averages exceeded these 95% limits. Cembrowski, Chandler, and Westgard used computer simulations of the SMAC analyzer to evaluate the AOP quality control procedure.[10] Systematic error was simulated and the proportion of occasions that the patient average was outside its error limits was determined. Power functions were generated by plotting these proportions against the magnitude of error.

These power functions demonstrated that there are 5 important parameters which should be considered when an AOP quality control system is implemented. In order of decreasing importance they are: (1) the ratio of the standard deviation of the patient population (s_p) to the standard deviation of the analytical method (s_a), expressed as s_p/s_a; (2) the number of patient results averaged (N_p); (3) the control limits and thus the probability of false rejection (P_{fr}); (4) the truncation limits for exclusion of patient data from being averaged; and (5) the population beyond the truncation limits.

In the absence of outliers, the influence of N_p and s_p/s_a on the error detection capabilities of AOP is demonstrated in Figure 7–3, families of power functions for glucose, potassium, creatinine, and sodium. Figure 7–3 shows that for increasing N_p, there is a marked increase in the probability of error detection (P_{ed}). For glucose, the P_{ed} of a 3s shift is 6, 17, 60, and 90% for N_p = 10, 20, 50, and 100, respectively. Small systematic errors are better detected with large N_p.

For constant N_p, the P_{ed} is inversely related to the ratio of s_p/s_a. As s_p/s_a approaches 1, the distribution of the patient population approximates that of the control observations with the average of only a few patient values having the power of one control. Table 7–7 lists s_p, s_a, and s_p/s_a for representative chemistry and hematology tests. The nomogram shown in Figure 7–4 provides the P_{ed} of detection of a $2s_a$ shift for various N_p and s_p/s_a. The P_{fr} for the nomogram is fixed at 1%. This nomogram can be used to determine the minimum number of patient data to be averaged for a $2s_a$ shift to be detected with a specific probability. For alkaline phosphatase, with a s_p/s_a of 9, a minimum of 200 patient values should be averaged for a $2s_a$ shift to be detected 60% of the time. For prothrombin time, with a s_p/s_a ratio of 3, a minimum of 22 patient values would have to be averaged to provide similar error detection capabilities.

Douville, Cembrowski, and Strauss have derived a formula for calculating the number of patient values which must be averaged to yield the error detection capabilities of control specimens.[13] If the power of the AOP procedure is to be roughly equivalent to the power offered by N_c control specimens, then the number of patient specimens (N_p) which must be analyzed is

$$N_p = 2 \times N_c \times (s_p/s_a)^2. \qquad \text{Eq. 7–3}$$

Conversely, when N_p patient data are averaged, the power of this control procedure is equal to N_c control specimens:

$$N_c = 0.5 \times N_p/(s_p/s_a)^2. \qquad \text{Eq. 7–4}$$

The estimate of N_p obtained from Equation 7–3 is the minimum number of patient values to be averaged. This estimate is usually too low because it corresponds to the optimal situation in which the population distribution is gaussian and outliers are not present (see below). In the presence of outliers or asymmetrical distributions, the number of pa-

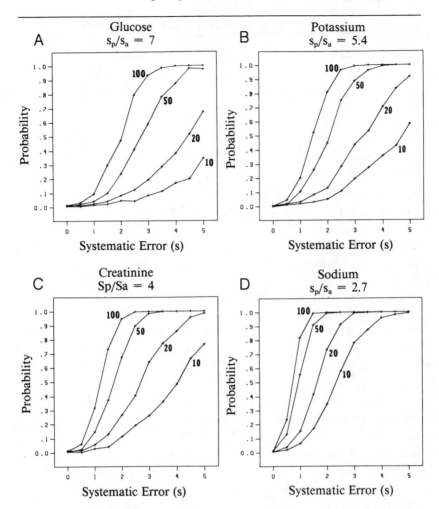

Figure 7–3 Power functions illustrating the effect of varying N_p and s_p/s_a. The probability of false rejection (P_{fr}) is fixed at 0.01.

Reproduced with permission. From Cembrowski GS, Chandler EP, Westgard JO: Assessment of "average of normals" quality control procedures and guidelines for implementation. Am J Clin Pathol 81:492-499, 1984.

tient values averaged should be increased to maintain acceptable error detection.

The effect of altering the *control limits* is shown in Figure 7–5. As the control limits are decreased from $\pm\ 3.09 \times s_p/\sqrt{N_p}$ to $\pm\ 2.58 \times$

Table 7-7   Values of s_p and s_a for various clinical laboratory tests.

Test	Mean	s_p	s_a	s_p/s_a
MCHC (g/dL)	35.1	0.83	0.5	1.7
Aspartate aminotransferase (U/L)	33	13.8	6.95	2.0
Calcium (mg/dL)	9.6	0.47	0.18	2.6
Sodium (mmol/L)	142.0	3.57	1.34	2.7
Total bilirubin (mg/dL)	0.4	0.19	0.066	2.9
Chloride (mmol/L)	103.6	3.46	1.21	2.9
Prothrombin time (s)	10	.45	.15	3.0
Partial thromboplastin time (s)	28	3.2	0.9	3.6
Albumin (g/dL)	3.9	0.44	0.12	3.7
Creatinine (mg/dL)	0.89	0.28	0.070	4.0
Total protein (g/dL)	6.9	0.62	0.13	4.8
Lactate dehydrogenase (U/L)	157	40.1	7.38	5.4
Potassium (mmol/L)	4.3	0.43	0.080	5.4
Gamma glutamyl transpeptidase (U/L)	31	20.0	3.15	6.3
Phosphorus (mg/dL)	3.6	0.66	0.096	6.9
Glucose (mg/L)	93.6	11.5	1.65	7.0
MCH (pg)	30.8	2.6	0.35	7.4
CO_2 (mmol/L)	25.2	6.59	0.84	7.8
Uric acid (mg/dL)	5.1	1.43	0.17	8.4
Cholesterol (mg/dL)	170	34.4	3.8	9.1
Alkaline phosphatase (U/L)	78	23.7	2.3	10
MCV (fL)	88	6.3	0.6	11
Urea nitrogen (mg/dL)	14.4	5.46	0.42	13
Hematocrit (%)	34.5	6.7	0.42	16
Red Cell Count ($\times 10^{12}$/L)	4.0	0.8	0.05	16
Hemoglobin (g/dL)	12	2.3	0.1	23

Note: The chemistry results were derived from SMAC, the coagulation results from the Coag-A-Mate X2, and the hematology results from the Coulter S + IV.

Reproduced with permission. From Cembrowski GS. Use of patient data for quality control. Clin Lab Med 6:715-733, 1986.

$s_p/\sqrt{N_p}$ to $\pm 1.96 \times s_p/\sqrt{N_p}$, the probability of false rejection increases from 0.2% to 1% to 5%, respectively. The power function curves are shifted to the left with smaller shifts detected with moderate probability. If the P_{fr} is fixed and N_p is increased, the control limits narrow and increase the probability of detecting small shifts, some of which

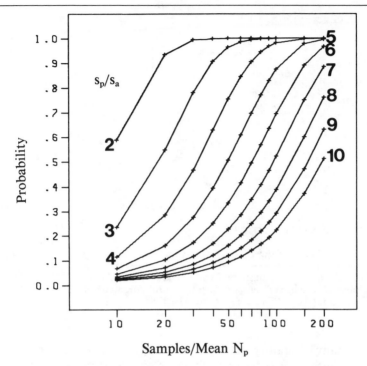

Figure 7–4 Nomogram illustrating the relationship between N_p, s_p/s_a, and the probability of detecting a $2s_a$ shift when the P_{fr} is 0.01.

Reproduced with permission. From Cembrowski GS, Chandler EP, Westgard JO: Assessment of "average of normals" quality control procedures and guidelines for implementation. Am J Clin Pathol 81:492-499, 1984.

may not be clinically significant (Figure 7–3). Thus, control limits may need to be widened to prevent the detection of shifts which are not important. Generally, control limits for the AOP procedure are selected in consideration of the power of the reference sample quality control procedure in use. If the reference sample procedure is weak, more sensitivity is required of the AOP procedure, and vice versa.

In the absence of outlying populations, the effects of varying the truncation limits are predictable; they are shown in Figure 7–6. As would be expected, there is little difference between averaging all the data and excluding any data outside the $3.09s_p$ or $2.58s_p$ limits. Only when the percentage of data excluded from averaging approaches 5% (using the $1.96s_p$ truncation limits) is there a moderate decrease in power with the curves shifting to the right.

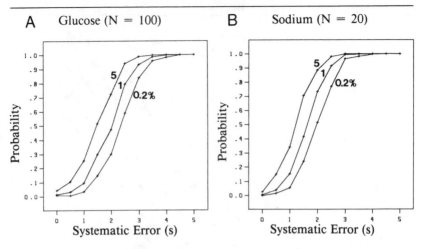

Figure 7–5 Effect of the P_{fr} on power functions.

Reproduced with permission. From Cembrowski GS, Chandler EP, Westgard JO: Assessment of "average of normals" quality control procedures and guidelines for implementation. Am J Clin Pathol 81:492-499, 1984.

For many laboratory tests, the frequency of outliers from the central distribution is high. The power function curves demonstrating the effects of s_p/s_a, N_p, control, and truncation limits were generated with the assumption that the patient data had no outliers. Simulations of distributions with *outlying populations* indicate that the power of tests with high s_p/s_a decreases dramatically with increasing proportions of outliers. There is lesser degradation in the power for tests with low s_p/s_a (Figure 7–7). When there are many outliers ($> 5\%$), narrow limits ($2.5s_p$) should be used to exclude them. Wide truncation limits ($3.0s_p$) should be considered when few outliers ($< 5\%$) are present.

Setup of an AOP procedure is not trivial. The following steps are required:

1. Collect consecutive patient data over several weeks and plot a frequency histogram of the data.

2. Characterize the patient population by using the data within the central region to calculate the mean and standard deviation (s_p).

3. Determine s_a from a control product whose mean concentration is close to the patient mean.

4. Estimate N_p from Equation 7–3 or from the nomogram based on s_p/s_a and the probability of detecting a shift of $2s_a$ or ΔSE_c.

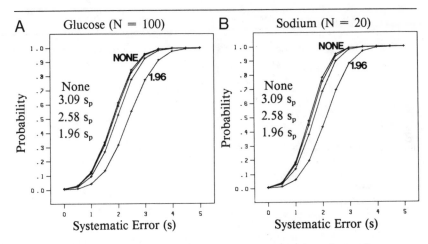

Figure 7-6 Effect of truncation limits on power functions for patient populations without outliers ($P_{fr} = 0.01$).

Reproduced with permission. From Cembrowski GS, Chandler EP, Westgard JO: Assessment of "average of normals" quality control procedures and guidelines for implementation. Am J Clin Pathol 81:492-499, 1984.

5. Select truncation limits.

6. Select the control limits so that the P_{fr} is no more than 1%.

7. Widen the control limits if probability of detecting small errors is too large.

The AOP quality control procedure has been applied to endocrinology assays by Douville et al.[13] The s_p/s_a ratios of various endocrinology assays done at the Hospital of the University of Pennsylvania are shown in Table 7-8. Because the thyroid hormones exhibited low s_p/s_a ratios, consistent with high error detection capabilities, the authors monitored the exponentially smoothed averages of patient thyroxine, triiodothyronine uptake, and free thyroid index data. They concluded that AOP can detect clinically important trends in patient data which can be missed by reference sample quality control. They found that AOP can be used to differentiate between analytical shifts (resulting in shifted patient average and control ranges) and deterioration in the control material (resulting in the usual patient average but shifted control ranges).

Douville has used AOP to monitor a general chemistry analyzer prospectively and adjust its calibration. Figure 7-8 illustrates some of

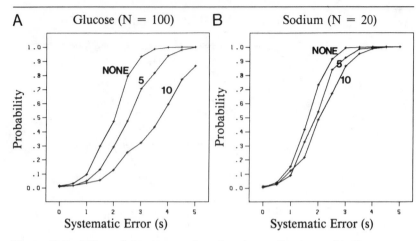

Figure 7-7 Effect of percentage of outliers immediately outside the truncation limits of 2.58 s_p. ($P_{fr} = 0.01$). Percentage of population outside truncation limits: 0%, 5%, 7%.

Reproduced with permission. From Cembrowski GS, Chandler EP, Westgard JO: Assessment of "average of normals" quality control procedures and guidelines for implemenation. Am J Clin Pathol 81:492-499, 1984.

his data, the AOP of sequential sodium data averaged by 2 different exponential smoothing constants, $\alpha = 0.3$ and $\alpha = 0.01$ (corresponding to averaging of approximately 6 and 199 observations, respectively). The exponentially smoothed sodiums show a decrease in the patient sodiums of approximately 6 mmol/L. This excursion is far more conspicuous when the sodium data are smoothed with $\alpha = 0.01$ than with $\alpha = 0.3$. Only one of the low-level control results is outside its error limits during this decrease of patient sodiums. Further evaluations of AOP are required before its true utility in the clinical laboratory is determined. In the future, optimized AOP procedures should become more useful for instrument monitoring as fewer and fewer controls are analyzed relative to the number of patient specimens.

Patient Red Cell Indices for Multichannel Hematology Instruments

Table 7-7 shows the s_p, s_a, and s_p/s_a for the red cell parameters provided by the Coulter multichannel hematology counter. This instrument measures the red cell count (RBC), hemoglobin (Hgb), and mean corpuscular volume (MCV) directly, and from these 3 parameters calculates the hematocrit (RBC × MCV), mean corpuscular

Table 7-8   Values of s_p and s_a for various endocrinology assays.

Test	Truncation Limits	s_p	s_a	s_p/s_a
T4 (ug/dL)	4–13	2.03	0.35	5.8
T3u	0.85–1.25	0.094	0.035	2.7
FTI	4–13	2.00	0.45	4.4
TSH (mU/L)	0–10	2.16	0.40	5.4
Prolactin (ug/L)	0–60	14.9	1.07	14
LH (U/L)	2–30	7.09	2.57	2.8
FSH (U/L)	0–25	5.2	1.94	2.7
Vitamin B12 (ng/L)	80–1000	208	45	4.6
Folate (ug/L)	2–13	2.49	0.31	8.0
Cortisol (ug/dL)	4–36	7.68	1.03	7.5
Estradiol (ng/L)	0–600	151	19.8	7.6
Testosterone (ng/dL)	15–110	20	6.2	3.2

Reproduced with permission. From Cembrowski GS: Use of patient data for quality control. Clin Lab Med 6:715-733, 1986.

hemoglobin or MCH (Hgb/RBC), and mean corpuscular hemoglobin concentration or MCHC (Hgb/(RBC $\times$ MCV)). The very low value of s_p/s_a for MCHC, approximately 2, indicates that relatively few (10 to 20) patient MCHC values would have to be averaged to detect a shift of $2s_a$ (See Figure 7-4). Conversely, at least 200 MCVs would have to be averaged for a $2s_a$ shift in MCV to be detected with a P_{ed} of at least 0.5.

The use of average patient red cell indices for quality control was advocated in the early 1960s,[14] and it gained popularity in the mid 1970s after Bull and coworkers recommended a novel technique for averaging the indices.[15] With this averaging technique, the new Bull's average is set to the last Bull's average plus the average deviation of the batch of red cell indices from the last Bull's average. The smoothing technique and its performance characteristics are presented in detail in Chapter 9.

MULTIVARIATE (INTERPARAMETRIC) CHECKS OF PATIENT DATA

The error detection capabilities of the red cell indices MCH and MCHC arise from the close association of the directly measured parameters RBC, Hgb, and MCV. Large random or systematic errors in

155

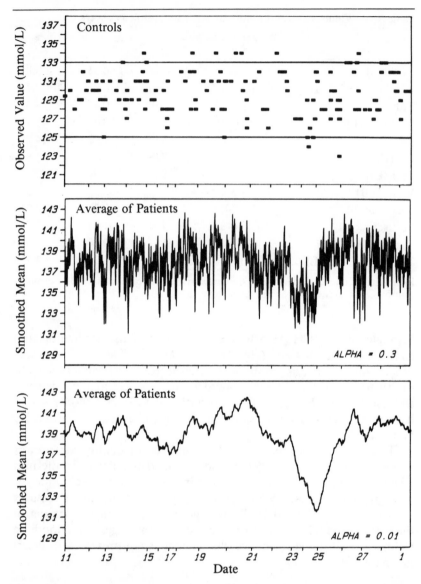

Figure 7–8 Exponentially smoothed mean of patient sodium data obtained by averaging consecutive ASTRA sodium data with $\alpha = 0.01$ (bottom) and with $\alpha = 0.3$ (middle). The top frame shows the sodium quality control data for the low level control.

(Data courtesy of Pierre Douville.)

these directly measured tests cause improbable MCH or MCHC values for individual patient specimens. Reanalysis of patient specimens with outlying indices can detect these large isolated errors. Smaller systematic errors can be detected by monitoring the average of MCH, MCHC, and MCV. Certain closely related biochemical parameters can be used for quality control in much the same way as the red cell indices. Van Kampen has used the term *interparametric quality control* to refer to the quality control which evaluates the concentrations of analytes which have a close relationship.[16] Two examples of relationships used in interparametric quality control are described in this section—the anion gap and the Henderson-Hasselbalch equation.

Anion Gap

The anion gap is usually calculated from the difference between Na^+ concentration and the sum of Cl^- and CO_2^- concentrations. Significant deviations of individual anion gaps from the average value of 11 to 12 mmol/L are usually due to disease, but less often may be due to laboratory error in Na^+, Cl^-, or CO_2^-. The quality control practice of reanalyzing patient specimens with abnormal anion gaps is common. Cembrowski et al have studied its performance characteristics by use of a computer simulation model of an electrolyte analyzer.[12] Even in the presence of large analytical errors ($3s_a$ to $5s_a$), the probability of detecting an anion gap greater than 20 or less than 4 mmol/L was very low when a healthy population was sampled. More often, especially in tertiary care hospitals, abnormal anion gaps are not caused by analytical error, but are truly abnormal.

The average of serial anion gaps can be used as a more specific indicator of instrument systematic error.[12] Moderate to large shifts ($>$ $2s_a$ shifts in Na^+ or Cl^-) can be detected by comparing the averages of consecutive anion gaps, 8 at a time, to the 99% confidence limits for the anion gap mean (7.5–13.5 mmol/L). To avoid known bias, patient specimens known to have low or high gaps should be excluded from averaging.

Subsequent work evaluated the use of average patient anion gaps for the detection of systematic error in the Beckman ASTRA (SmithKline Beckman, Brea, CA) electrolyte analyzer, an instrument which had a tendency to generate low anion gap values.[17] A total of 36 runs of 8 patient specimens with low anion gap averages ($<$ 7.5 mmol/L) were reanalyzed after appropriate recalibration and/or maintenance. Thirty-one of the 36 groups had significant changes in either Na^+ (9 groups, $\Delta Na^+ = +1.5$ mmol/L), Cl^- (14 groups, $\Delta Cl^- = -1.8$

mmol/L), or in both Na$^+$ and Cl$^-$ (8 groups, ΔNa$^+$ = +1.2 mmol/L; ΔCl$^-$ = -0.9 mmol/L). Figure 7-9 shows the change in the average and maximum Na$^+$ and Cl$^-$, after reanalysis of the sets of patient specimens. Overall, the average magnitude of the error detected was small. When combined errors were present which increased or decreased the anion gap, eg a decreased Na$^+$ and an increased Cl$^-$, the size of the error detected in individual patient Na$^+$ and Cl$^-$ values was even smaller. Because of the high sensitivity to small combined errors, the average of anion gaps can be used as an early indicator of drift and the need for corrective action before the development of significant errors.

The average of anion gaps, like the average of red cell indices, has limitations. It cannot detect random error. Similarly, negative or positive shifts in both Na$^+$ and Cl$^-$ or Na$^+$ and CO$_2^-$ cannot be detected. The anion gap calculation is best used in conjunction with standard quality control procedures, such as the multirule approach, to indicate a need for instrument maintenance or recalibration. Followup of single anion gaps is usually not needed unless the analytical system is overly sensitive to bromide interference.[18] If this is the case, then specimens with anion gaps less than 4 mmol/L should have their chloride reanalyzed on an instrument not affected by bromide. Unfortunately, many laboratories do not have alternative chloride methodologies.

Acid-base Balance

The relationship between pH, CO$_2$, and pCO$_2$ is expressed by the Henderson-Hasselbalch equation:

$$pH = 6.1 + \log ([CO_2]/.03 \, pCO_2) . \qquad \text{Eq. 7-5}$$

Laboratories which measure blood gases and electrolytes side by side can evaluate the validity of the pCO$_2$ and pH measured by the blood gas instrument by comparing the CO$_2$ calculated from the Henderson-Hasselbalch equation to the CO$_2$ measured by the electrolyte analyzer. Van Kampen correlated the calculated CO$_2^-$ of approximately 1000 blood gas analyses to the measured CO$_2^-$.[16] He found discordant results for approximately 12% of the comparisons. Upon remeasurement, 8% of the discrepancies were due to the pCO$_2$ determination; 3.5% were in pH, and 0.5% in CO$_2^-$. While comparison of the calculated and measured CO$_2$ is an accepted quality control practice at some institutions, its popularity is waning as blood gas services are being placed closer to critical care areas and away from the central laboratory. Performance of blood gas and electrolyte testing in different laboratories complicates the CO$_2$ correlations and any subsequent instrument in-

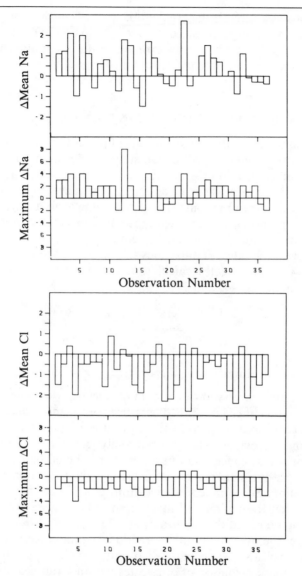

Figure 7–9 Changes in average and maximum sodium and chloride after 36 sets of 8 patient specimens were reanalyzed following either recalibration or system maintenance. Note difference in scales for the average and maximum changes.

terventions. Two trends may make this quality control practice more prevalent, the emergence of computer systems (either laboratory or hospitalwide) that maintain the patient's entire laboratory database, and placement of electrolyte instruments in the critical care laboratories.

DUPLICATE ANALYSIS OF PATIENT SPECIMENS

In Chapter 2, the duplicate analysis of patient specimens was used to determine a method's within-run standard deviation for "real" patient specimens (in contrast to control materials). Also, range rules (described in Chapter 3) can be applied to the ranges of the duplicates to detect within-run random error. Since some analytical procedures, eg, radioimmunoassay, are normally run in duplicate, they present the opportunity for more "free" quality control.

Limits for the range of duplicates can be derived from the standard deviation of the duplicates (calculation shown in Chapter 2) according to Equations 7–6, 7–7, and 7–8:[19,20]

$$\text{Limit for } R_{0.025} = s_{\text{duplicates}} \times 3.17. \qquad \text{Eq. 7–6}$$

$$\text{Limit for } R_{0.01} = s_{\text{duplicates}} \times 3.64. \qquad \text{Eq. 7–7}$$

$$\text{Limit for } R_{0.001} = s_{\text{duplicates}} \times 4.65. \qquad \text{Eq. 7–8}$$

Range rules with a very low P_{fr} should be selected when there are more than 3 or 4 specimens per run. These tests of the individual ranges of duplicates are more useful for detecting individual poor duplicates than for judging the overall quality of an analytical run. Rejections from specimens whose concentrations are extreme should be regarded cautiously, since the standard deviation is usually a function of analyte concentration. Some independence from concentration effects is offered by calculation of range limits in terms of coefficients of variation, and testing ranges of the duplicates as CVs.

Tests of the overall within-run random variation based on patient duplicates can also be accomplished with the chi-square test of the overall standard deviation of duplicates within a run against the historical within-run standard deviation of duplicates (see Chapter 3). Again, interpretation must be cautious when there are patient specimens with extreme concentrations.

When the analyst is not informed of the identity of the duplicates, the procedure is referred to as "blind." Application of control limits to the differences between blind duplicates has been proposed as a quality control procedure which avoids the bias of known controls. Grannis and Statland[21] and Bokelund, Winkel, and Statland[22] give procedures for blind duplicates, and some laboratory information systems have provision for blind duplicates. When extra duplicates are run, it is "extra" testing, not "free" like some other quality control procedures utilizing patient data. Weinberg and Barnett[23] found that operator knowledge of the identity of the specimens made no difference in their analysis. The authors' experience has been similar. There are operational problems with blind duplicate quality control procedures, as well. The duplicate specimen must have a plausible false identity. The plebotomist must have a method of identifying the blind duplicate to avoid mixups of the duplicates. If the specimen with the false identity has a test result exceeding a panic value, much time and emotion may be spent trying to inform appropriate nursing personnel about a test result which is life threatening to a fictitious patient. Eliminating operator bias just may not be cost-effective. Effective supervision is preferable.

PATIENT SAMPLE COMPARISONS

Some laboratories can routinely measure specific analytes by more than 1 method. Regular analysis of the same specimen(s) by the available methods (patient specimen comparisons) allows a check of the methods. For example, in addition to measuring albumin concentration directly, many laboratories can determine albumin concentration electrophoretically as part of the protein electrophoresis. The directly measured albumin can be compared to the electrophoretically determined albumin with differences indicating problems in one of the analytical systems. Patient sample comparisons are used to test agreement between analytical methods, independent of control materials, for example, agreement of enzyme results between a STAT instrument and a screening instrument. Typically, 2 or 3 patient specimens are selected to be run on both methods, and the resulting individual differences are compared to statistically derived limits.

Lunetzky and Cembrowski have studied the performance of some "control rules" for interpreting the differences.[24] Standard deviations of the differences were calculated as standard deviations of duplicates (assumes no bias). Optimal performance was obtained when 3 specimens are analyzed by both methods, with rejection being defined by 2 of the 3 specimens exceeding 2.5s limits $(2 \text{ of } 3)_{2.5s}$. The P_{ed} for detecting a bias of 2s between the methods was only 0.31, but use of 1_{3s} and $(2 \text{ of } 3)_{2s}$ rules resulted in an excessive P_{fr}.

When bias already exists between methods X and Y, control limits for the $(2 \text{ of } 3)_{2.5s}$ rule must be calculated using the bias and standard deviation of differences (s_d) from 40 or more patient comparison specimens:

$$\text{bias} = \bar{Y} - \bar{X}, \qquad \text{Eq. 7-9}$$

$$s_d = \sqrt{[\Sigma(y_i - x_i - \text{bias})^2/(N - 1)]}, \qquad \text{Eq. 7-10}$$

where N is the number of patient specimens.

$$\text{Limits} = \text{bias} \pm 2.5s_d. \qquad \text{Eq. 7-11}$$

FUTURE IMPLEMENTATIONS OF PATIENT DATA ALGORITHMS

As automated analyzers have become increasingly precise, repetitious analysis of commercial controls has become less efficient as a quality control procedure, and less cost effective. Increasingly, quality control of the analyzers will be accomplished through instrument diagnostics and algorithms utilizing patient data. These control procedures add negligible cost to patient care, and provide control during the periods when control materials are not being run. For most analytes, control procedures utilizing patient data have not been optimized as well as the procedures utilizing control materials. Even after they are better optimized, the LIS and HIS must undergo extensive development before these procedures can be introduced into the routine operation of the laboratory.

REFERENCES

1. Baer DM: Critical values for drug levels. Med Lab Obs 14(8):46-47, 1982.
2. Clevenger RR: A protocol for verifying critical values. Med Lab Obs 17(5):72-76, 1985.
3. Lindberg DAB: Collection, evaluation and transmission of hospital laboratory data. Methods Inf Med 6:97-107, 1967.
4. Nosanchuk JS, Gottmann AW: CUMS and delta checks. Am J Clin Pathol 62:707-712, 1974.
5. Wheeler LA, Sheiner LB: A clinical evaluation of various delta check methods. Clin Chem 27:5-9, 1981.
6. Wheeler LA, Sheiner LB: Delta check tables for the Technicon SMA 6 continuous-flow analyzer. Clin Chem 23:216-219, 1977.

7. Sheiner, LB, Wheeler LA, Moore JK: The performance of delta check methods. Clin Chem 25:2034-2037, 1979.

8. Iizuka Y, Kume H, Kitamura M: Multivariate delta check method for detecting specimen mix-up. Clin Chem 28:2244-2248, 1982.

9. Hoffmann RG, Waid NE: The "average of normals" method of quality control. Am J Clin Pathol 43:134-141, 1965.

10. Cembrowski GS, Chandler EP, Westgard JO: Assessment of "average of normals" quality control procedures and guidelines for implementation. Am J Clin Pathol 81:492-499, 1984.

11. Cembrowski GS, Westgard JO: Quality control of multichannel hematology analyzers: evaluation of Bull's algorithm. Am J Clin Pathol 83:337-345, 1985.

12. Cembrowski GS, Westgard JO, Kurtycz DFI: Use of anion gap for the quality control of electrolyte analyzers. Am J Clin Pathol 79:688-696, 1983.

13. Douville P, Cembrowski GS, Strauss J: Evaluation of the average of patients, application to endocrine assays. Clin Chim Acta 167:173-185, 1987.

14. Dorsey DB: Quality control in hematology. Am J Clin Pathol 40:457-464, 1963.

15. Bull BS, Elashoff RM, Heilbron AC, Couperus J: A study of various estimators for the derivation of quality control procedures from patient erythrocyte indices. Am J Clin Pathol 61:473-481, 1974.

16. Van Kampen EJ: Throwing a curve at laboratory error. Diag Med 3:54-61, 1980.

17. Bockelman HW, Cembrowski GS, Kurtycz DFI, et al: Quality control of electrolyte analyzers, evaluation of the anion gap average. Am J Clin Pathol 81:219-223, 1984.

18. Elin RJ, Robertson EA, Johnson E: Bromide interferes with determination of chloride by each of four methods. Clin Chem 27:778-779, 1981.

19. Davies OW, Goldsmith PL: Statistical Methods in Research and Production, ed 4. Longman, New York, 1984, pp 450-451.

20. Westgard JO, Groth T, Aronnson T, Falk H, de Verdier C-H: Performance characteristics of rules for internal quality control: probabilities for false rejection and error detection. Clin Chem 23:1857-1867, 1977.

21. Grannis GF, Statland BE: Monitoring the quality of laboratory measurements. In Henry JB, ed, Clinical Diagnosis and Management by Laboratory Methods. Saunders, Philadelphia, 1979, pp 2049-2068.

22. Bokelund H, Winkel P, Statland BE: Factors contributing to intraindividual variation of serum constituents: 3. Use of randomized duplicates to evaluate sources of analytic error. Clin Chem 20:1507-1512, 1974.

23. Weinberg M, Barnett RN: Absence of analytic bias in a quality control program. Am J Clin Pathol 38:468-472, 1962.

24. Lunetzky ES, Cembrowski GS: Optimized guidelines for inter-instrument validation. Clin Chem 33:909, 1987.

25. Whitehurst P, DiSilvio TV, Boyadjian G: Evaluation of discrepancies in patients' results—an aspect of computer-assisted quality control. Clin Chem 21:87-92, 1975.

26. Ladenson JH: Patients as their own controls: use of the computer to identify "laboratory error". Clin Chem 21:1648-1653, 1975.

27. Sher PP: Computer-assisted quality control in clinical chemistry. Clin Chem 23:871, 1977.

CHAPTER EIGHT

Design of Control Procedures to Meet Quality Specifications

This chapter addresses some of the practical aspects of setting up a quality control program. It considers control materials, control ranges, and the application of control procedures to generic laboratory analyses, as well as to specific clinical chemistry analyses. Guidelines are presented for designing control procedures so that the frequency of medically significant errors does not exceed allowable defect rates.

CONTROL MATERIALS

One of the first and most important steps in establishing a quality control program is the selection of appropriate control material. Long-term stability, sample-to-sample consistency, safety, and the ability to simulate patient specimens constitute the quality requirements of control materials.[1-4] Stability during the shelf storage and the use of the control material is paramount. Stability should be evaluated to verify that the day-to-day precision of control results is similar to that of patient specimens. Control products which yield high standard deviations compared to patient specimens should be rejected.

The control material should be packaged in a size which minimizes waste. Vial-to-vial consistency after reconstitution or thawing will minimize the control material's contribution to the between-run variation. The material should be able to tolerate slight differences in reconstitution and handling. The control material should be safe, ie, it should not contain reactive chemicals or infectious agents.

The control material's behavior during sampling and analysis should mimic a patient specimen as closely as possible. While the behavior of patient specimens is better simulated by human-based rather than bovine-based materials, human-based materials are infectious, more expensive, and may not be available in sufficient quantities to make large control pools. For some analytes, the control material source or preparation can cause differences between the analytical behavior of the control material and that of patient specimens.[2] For example, control sera of animal origin may not be satisfactory for albumin or some enzymes. Plug lyophilized control materials are frequently more turbid than patient specimens. "Liquid" controls stabilized with ethylene glycol are not acceptable specimens for osmolality. Other stability and reproducibility issues were discussed in Chapter 6.

The concentration of each analyte should be near the analyte's medical decision level; several materials may be required if there are multiple decision levels. Table 5–1 is a starting point for selecting desirable control material concentrations. For example, sodium requires 2 different materials, 1 at the near hyponatremic level, approximately 130 mmol/L and 1 in near hypernatremic level, approximately 150 to 160 mmol/L. Often it is not necessary to control at each decision level concentration, but the range of control concentrations should at least span the range of decision level concentrations.

While tri-level controls are popular, many analytes require only 2 levels. For example, various immunoassay control systems employ 3 different concentrations of analyte. Frequently 1 or more of these concentrations is not near a medical decision level. For example, 1 series of vitamin B-12 controls has concentrations of 200, 1000, and 1700 pg/mL. The vitamin B-12 control at 1700 pg/mL provides little relevant information. If 3 controls per run are required for an acceptable P_{ed}, a second control replicate should be analyzed whose concentration is near a decision level, say the 200 pg/mL control. This approach eliminates the variation introduced by the third control material itself. Haven has aptly stated,[5] "Routine use of tri-level quality control materials serves largely to increase manufacturer sales of control products and to slightly increase reagent utilization." For reasons of economy, it is common practice to use the same control product for a group of tests, such as a group of immunoassays or therapeutic drug methods; thus, some compromise on concentrations is inevitable.

ESTABLISHING CONTROL RANGES

For control rules to work effectively in a laboratory, control ranges must be customized for each laboratory. The next sections describe how new control materials are introduced and how their analytical values are transformed into statistically appropriate control ranges.

"Breaking In" New Controls

Optimally, control data should be collected from at least 20 runs from different days before control ranges are calculated. The annual or biannual process of "crossing over" from nearly outdated lots of control material to new lots can be traumatic because the period for concurrently analyzing the new and old lots is often less than 1 month. There tends to be confusion in recording control results during this "break in" period, especially if the old and new materials are from the same manufacturer and their analyte concentrations are similar.

Once the new materials are used exclusively, apparent false rejection problems may arise with 1 or more of the newly established control ranges, especially when many analytes are involved. The ranges may be too narrow due to 2 factors: limited statistical sample and underestimation of the long-term variation.

When a standard deviation is estimated from small numbers of control observations, the true standard deviation is not known exactly because of the limited statistical sample. Confidence limits for the true standard deviation can be calculated around an estimated standard deviation in a manner analogous to confidence limits around an observed mean. Natrella and others have provided factors for calculating these limits.[6-8] For example, if there are 21 observations (20 degrees of freedom) for the standard deviation, the 95% confidence limits are located at 0.75s and 1.42s.[7] As the number of observations increases, the confidence limits around the estimated standard deviation shrink; for 101 observations, the 95% confidence limits are at 0.88s and 1.16s.

Ross has estimated that the standard deviation calculated from 1 month's data is 80% of the total standard deviation and the standard deviation calculated from 6 months' data is 99% of the total standard deviation.[9] This observation suggests that day-to-day variation is underestimated during the break in period.

It is common practice to obtain several results each day for each analyte and control material combination in order to have more observations for calculation of the mean and standard deviation. The incorporation of more than 1 replicate per day into the calculation of the standard deviation causes underestimation of the standard deviation when it is calculated according to Equation 2-2.[10,11] Equation 2-2 is accurate when single daily observations are incorporated. The underestimation may become severe as the number of replicates per day increases and the number of days decreases below 20 days, especially for methods with $s_b > s_w$. The next section demonstrates how a statistical procedure, analysis of variance, can be used to determine re-

167

alistic estimates of the between- and within-day standard deviations as well as the total standard deviation.

Analysis of Variance (ANOVA) Procedure and Calculations

It is a common misconception that preliminary control ranges can be derived from the standard deviation of 20 control measurements gathered over a period considerably shorter than 20 days. If multiple observations are collected each day, the standard deviation of all the observations will reflect both the within-day and between-day standard deviations. If the within-day component of standard deviation is much smaller than the between-day component, the resulting total standard deviation will be erroneously small because the between-day variation is underestimated. Use of control limits based on this artefactually small standard deviation will result in rejection of excess numbers of analytical runs without increased analytical error.

If multiple control observations are gathered daily, accurate estimates of the standard deviation can be obtained with analysis of variance (ANOVA) calculations. The ANOVA technique separates the within-run, between-run, and between-day components of variation and recombines them, giving each its proper weight in the calculation of the total standard deviation. Bauer and Kennedy and the National Committee for Clinical Laboratory Standards (NCCLS) have published procedures for estimating total standard deviations by the ANOVA technique.[10,12,13]

ANOVA calculations usually require that the number of control specimens analyzed in every run and the number of runs per day remain constant. The NCCLS document contains worksheets and formulae for 2 runs per day, with controls assayed in duplicate within each run. The worksheets provide a convenient guide for the manual calculation of the total standard deviation. Modifications are provided for 1 run per day. Figure 8–1 shows an ANOVA computer program based on the NCCLS document which was developed by one of the authors. The program is written in BASIC and can be run on virtually any microcomputer. The program combines between-run and between-day variations as s_b^2 (see Chapter 2), assumes 1 run per day, and allows the user to specify the number of replicates to be analyzed within the run. An example of input data and program output is shown in Figure 8–2.

Treatment of Outliers

During the breaking in of a new control, there may be outlying observations for which there is no apparent cause. Until a large number

```
10 REM ANOVA PRECISION EVALUATION EXPERIMENT FOR ONE RUN PER DAY
20 REM  AND UP TO A MAXIMUM OF FIVE (5) TESTS PER RUN
30 REM  PROGRAM WRITTEN BY J. TYVOLL - MODIFIED BY P. UPHAM
40 REM  EQUATIONS FROM NCCLS EP5; NEGATIVE DAY-TO-DAY CORRECTED
50 REM  VARIANCE SET TO ZERO ******************************
60 LPRINT CHR$(27)"N"CHR$(12)
70 DIM D(50,5),SW(50),MEAN(50):X=14
80 PRINT TAB(10)"****** PRECISION EVALUATION EXPERIMENT ******":PRINT
100 INPUT "ENTER ANALYTE: -- ",A$:PRINT
130 INPUT "ENTER DESCRIPTION: -- ",B$:PRINT
160 INPUT "ENTER # REPLICATIONS PER RUN: -- ",T:PRINT:PRINT
200 I=1:PRINT
220 PRINT "FOR DAY "I" ENTER DATA - TYPE -999 IF NO MORE DATA IS TO BE ENTERED"
230 FOR J=1 TO T:PRINT
250  PRINT "REP. # "J
260  INPUT D(I,J)
270  IF D(I,J)=-999 THEN GOTO 320
280 NEXT J
290 D=I:I=I+1
310 PRINT:GOTO 220
320 CHK$="OFF":PRINT
340 PRINT"*** PRINTER SHOULD BE -ON LINE- FOR DATA REVIEW ***":PRINT
360 INPUT "END OF DATA ENTRY: REVIEW/EDIT DATA (YES/NO)?",R$
380 IF R$="NO" OR R$="N" GOTO 680:IF CHK$="OFF" THEN GOTO 410
400 LPRINT CHR$(140)
410 LPRINT TAB(17);"ANOVA PRECISION EVALUATION USING ONE RUN PER DAY":LPRINT
430 LPRINT:LPRINT "ANALYTE: "A$:LPRINT "DESCRIPTION: "B$:LPRINT:LPRINT
435 LPRINT TAB(5)"DAY";
437 FOR Z=1 TO T
440  LPRINT TAB(X)"REP. "Z;
445  X=X+10:NEXT Z:LPRINT
450 X=15:FOR I=1 TO D:LPRINT
460  LPRINT TAB(6) I;
470   FOR J=1 TO T
480    LPRINT TAB(X) D(I,J);
485    X=X+10
490   NEXT J
492  X=15
493 NEXT I
520 PRINT:INPUT "DO YOU WISH TO CHANGE VALUES (YES/NO)?",R$
540 IF R$="NO" OR R$="N" THEN LPRINT CHR$(12):PRINT:GOTO 360
560 LPRINT:LPRINT "*** THIS DATA SET INCLUDES INCORRECT VALUES - DISCARD ***"
580 LPRINT CHR$(12):PRINT:INPUT "INPUT DAY #, REP. #, AND THE NEW VALUE -- ",I,J,N
610 PRINT:PRINT " DAY "I"  REP. # "J
630 PRINT:PRINT "*** CORRECTED DATA VALUE = "N
650 PRINT:D(I,J)=N
660 CHK$="ON"
670 PRINT:GOTO 520
```

Figure 8–1A Part 1 of BASIC program for ANOVA calculation of standard deviation when more than one control replicate is tested per day in one run per day.

of observations are accumulated, it is difficult to judge whether these outliers are representative of the control population. Tests for outliers should be used to exclude outlying observations, but these tests should be "conservative" and not exclude excess numbers of observations, since the number of control observations is limited. Elimination of

169

```
680 GSUM=0
690 FOR I=1 TO D
700   SUM=0
710   FOR J=1 TO T
720     SUM=SUM+D(I,J)
730   NEXT J
740   MEAN(I)=SUM/T:GSUM=GSUM+MEAN(I)
760 NEXT I
770 GMEAN=GSUM/D:SUM=0
790 FOR I=1 TO D
800   TEMP=(MEAN(I)-GMEAN):SUM=SUM+TEMP^2
820 NEXT I
830 BB=SUM/(D-1):B=SQR(BB):SSUM=0
860 FOR I=1 TO D
870   TEMP=0
880   FOR J=1 TO T
890     D2=D(I,J)-MEAN(I):D2=D2^2:TEMP=TEMP+D2:SSUM=SSUM+D2
930   NEXT J
940   SW(I)=TEMP/(T-1)
950 NEXT I
960 BTERM=D*(T-1):SWR1=SSUM/BTERM:SWR=SQR(SWR1):ST=BB+((T-1)/T)*SWR1
1000 ST=SQR(ST):SDDVAR=BB-(SWR1/T):SDD=SQR(SDDVAR)
1030 LPRINT CHR$(140):LPRINT
1050 LPRINT TAB(17);"ANOVA PRECISION EVALUATION FOR ONE RUN PER DAY":LPRINT
1070 LPRINT:LPRINT "NO. REPLICATES PER RUN = "T;TAB(33);"ANALYTE: "A$
1080 LPRINT "DESCRIPTION: "B$:LPRINT:LPRINT
1140 LPRINT " DAY #"TAB(15)"RUN MEAN"TAB(55)"RUN VARIANCE"
1150 LPRINT" -----"TAB(15)"---------"TAB(55)"------------"
1160 FOR I=1 TO D
1170   LPRINT TAB(3)I;:LPRINT USING "###.###";TAB(16);MEAN(I);TAB(58);SW(I)
1180 NEXT I
1200 LPRINT TAB(15) "---------" TAB(55)"------------":LPRINT
1210 LPRINT " GRAND MEAN = ";:LPRINT USING "###.###";GMEAN;TAB(40);
1215 LPRINT "S.D. OF DAILY MEANS = ";:LPRINT USING "###.###";B:LPRINT:LPRINT
1220 LPRINT:LPRINT TAB(30)"STANDARD DEVIATION" TAB(53)"VARIANCE":LPRINT
1230 LPRINT TAB(15);"WITHIN RUN ";TAB(36);:LPRINT USING "###.###";SWR;TAB(54);SWR1
1240 LPRINT TAB(15);"BETWEEN RUN ";TAB(36);:LPRINT USING
                        "###.###";SDD;TAB(54);SDDVAR
1250 LPRINT TAB(35);"---------";TAB(53);"---------"
1330 LPRINT:LPRINT TAB(15);"TOTAL ";TAB(36);:LPRINT USING "###.###";ST;TAB(54);ST^2
1340 LPRINT CHR$(140);:LPRINT CHR$(12)
1360 INPUT "DO YOU WISH TO RUN ANOTHER SET OF DATA (YES/NO)?",R$
1380 IF R$="YES" OR R$="Y" GOTO 80:PRINT
1400 PRINT"**** END OF PRECISION EXPERIMENT ****"
1410 END
```

Figure 8–1B Part 2 of BASIC program for ANOVA calculation of standard deviation when more than one control replicate is tested per day in one run per day.

control results which are not true outliers will result in an artificially low standard deviation and control range. However, if true outliers are not eliminated, the standard deviation may be inflated, and the mean may be inaccurate. Either effect, the elimination of excess numbers of control observations, or the inclusion of outliers, will degrade the performance of quality control procedures.

Observations more than 3.0 or 3.5 standard deviations from the

NO. REPLICATES PER RUN = 2   ANALYTE: Glucose
DESCRIPTION: #1

DAY #	RUN MEAN	RUN VARIANCE
1	84.500	0.500
2	91.500	4.500
3	88.000	0.000
4	89.000	2.000
5	87.500	0.500
6	89.000	0.000
7	87.500	0.500
8	89.000	2.000
9	88.500	0.500
10	90.000	0.000
11	88.000	2.000
12	88.500	0.500
13	89.500	0.500
14	89.000	0.000
15	92.500	0.500
16	88.000	0.000
17	91.500	0.500
18	89.000	8.000
19	92.000	0.000
20	91.500	0.500

GRAND MEAN = 89.200   S.D. OF DAILY MEANS = 1.902

	STANDARD DEVIATION	VARIANCE
WITHIN RUN	1.072	1.150
BETWEEN RUN	1.744	3.041
TOTAL	2.047	4.191

ANALYTE: Glucose
DESCRIPTION: #1

DAY	REP. 1	REP. 2
1	85	84
2	90	93
3	88	88
4	88	90
5	88	87
6	89	89
7	87	88
8	88	90
9	89	88
10	90	90
11	89	87
12	88	89
13	90	89
14	89	89
15	92	93
16	88	88
17	92	91
18	91	87
19	92	92
20	91	92

Figure 8–2   (A) Example of replicate control data from 1 run per day evaluated with ANOVA and (B) a facsimile of output of ANOVA analysis.

mean (z-score > 3.0 or 3.5) are typically considered outliers.[7] Burnett has provided criteria for outlier identification for various sample sizes with 5% risk of incorrectly identifying an observation as an outlier.[8] When there are 20 observations, the criterion is 3.02; any observation more than 3.02s from the mean is considered an outlier. For 40, 60, 80, 100, and 200 observations, the criteria are 3.22, 3.33, 3.41, 3.47, 3.66, respectively. When an outlier is identified, the mean and standard deviation are recomputed after elimination of the outlier(s).

Regardless of how outliers are treated, their frequency should be carefully monitored because a high outlier frequency may indicate underlying problems with the analytical method, control material, or analyst technique. The entire analytical method, including control procedure, should be carefully investigated for causes of the outliers. More than 3 outliers per 100 observations is cause for serious concern about the method or control material.

It is even more important to avoid eliminating control results after the control material is in routine use. It is still common practice to retest a control if its result is between the mean $\pm$ 2s and mean $\pm$ 3s control limits, and to record the "good" result. This practice artificially narrows the control range. Even when a single control is analyzed, and the run is repeated because the control result falls in this range, the control result should still be recorded and used in statistical calculations unless a problem is recognized in the method independent of the control result.

SELECTING CONTROL PROCEDURES

The preceding chapters have shown that the determination of the appropriate control procedure for a given analytical method depends on the interaction among the inherent random error of the method, the medically allowable error, and the prevalence of errors which cause total error to exceed the allowable error. For example, if the medically allowable error, E_a, is less than the inherent random error of a method (1.96s or 2.58s for 95% and 99% limits, respectively), no amount of quality control can maintain total error below E_a. On the other hand, if the inherent random error is much less than E_a, and the prevalence, prev, of large errors is very small, an insensitive quality control procedure may be adequate to maintain errors below E_a 95% (or 99%) of the time. Quality control theory has not advanced sufficiently to state that a certain method with given values of allowable error, prevalence, and total standard deviation requires quality control procedure XYZ; however, it is now possible to calculate the probability of error detection required (for ΔSE_c and ΔRE_c) to maintain errors below E_a 95% or 99% of the time.

Westgard and Barry have shown how the percentage of results with errors exceeding E_a can be calculated from the above parameters, and have described some guidelines for designing cost-effective quality control procedures.[14] The following sections are based on their guidelines.

Estimating Medically Important Errors

Chapter 5 demonstrated the calculation of the critical random and critical systematic errors from E_a and the standard deviation. For a 95% limit of error (5% error rate), ΔRE_c is given by

$$\Delta RE_c = \frac{E_a}{1.96s_t}, \qquad \text{Eq. 8–1A}$$

where s_t represents the total standard deviation.

For a 99% limit of error (1% error rate), ΔRE_c is given by

$$\Delta RE_c = \frac{E_a}{2.58s_t}. \qquad \text{Eq. 8–1B}$$

If the calculated value of ΔRE_c is less than 1, then the defect rate of the analytical method already exceeds the maximum allowable rate.

The critical systematic error, ΔSE_c, also expressed in multiples of the long-term standard deviation, is given by Equation 8–2A for a 5% error rate:

$$\Delta SE_c = \frac{E_a}{s_t} - 1.65, \qquad \text{Eq. 8–2A}$$

and Equation 8–2B for a 1% error rate:

$$\Delta SE_c = \frac{E_a}{s_t} - 2.33. \qquad \text{Eq. 8–2B}$$

If the calculated value of ΔSE_c is less than 0.0, then the defect rate of the analytical method already exceeds the maximum allowable rate.

If the magnitude of the medically allowable error is not defined, Westgard recommends the critical random and systematic errors be set equal to twice the standard deviation.[14] Thus $\Delta RE_c = 2s_t$, and $\Delta SE_c = 2 s_t$.

Prevalence of Medically Important Errors

Accurate determination of the prevalence of medically important errors is difficult, as was shown in Chapter 5. If prevalence is low, accurate estimates can be provided only by assaying enough controls in each run to use rules having a sufficiently high P_{ed} to guarantee detecting errors exceeding ΔRE_c and ΔSE_c, and having a sufficiently low P_{fr} to avoid biasing the estimate of prevalence with false rejections. Even then, the magnitudes of the errors detected may not be known well enough to determine their medical importance. The prevalence of increased errors can be estimated from previous experience with the method if ΔRE_c and ΔSE_c are high enough to be detected by the quality control procedure in use. While most estimates of prevalence are simply educated guesses, they are essential in predicting the performance of control procedures.

Part of the prevalence of medically important errors arises from the method's inherent random error, since the inherent error causes some results to have errors exceeding E_a, as was shown in Chapter 5. The prevalence of medically important errors caused by the inherent random error increases as s_t increases relative to E_a. This relationship between prevalence and the ratio of E_a/s_t is demonstrated in Table 8–1. Since ΔRE_c and ΔSE_c are calculated from E_a/s_t, low values for ΔRE_c and ΔSE_c indicate high error prevalences.

Estimating the P_{ed} Required to Maintain an Acceptable Defect Rate

Westgard and Barry[14] have shown that the defect rate (DR) of an analytical process (percentage of results with errors exceeding E_a) is given by

$$DR = prev(1 - P_{ed}), \qquad \text{Eq. 8–3}$$

where prev is the prevalence of errors whose magnitudes exceed E_a. Equation 8–3 can be rearranged to yield the P_{ed} needed to maintain a chosen defect rate:

$$P_{ed} = \frac{prev - DR}{prev}. \qquad \text{Eq. 8–4}$$

If the prev $<$ DR, the required P_{ed} will be negative, and should be set to 0; no error detection is necessary. In effect, whenever the prev $<$ DR, a low P_{ed} is acceptable. Thus, quality control procedures optimized to provide low P_{fr} values should be used to avoid the cost of unnecessary false rejections.

Table 8–1   Prevalence of errors exceeding E_a.

$\dfrac{E_a}{s_t}$	Error Prevalence
1.90	0.057
1.96	0.050
2.00	0.046
2.10	0.036
2.20	0.028
2.30	0.021
2.40	0.016
2.50	0.012
2.58	0.010
2.60	0.009
2.70	0.007
2.80	0.005
2.90	0.004
3.00	0.003

Note: Prevalence due to inherent random error as a function of s_t and E_a, as derived from the gaussian distribution.

As prevalence increases, the P_{ed} must increase in order to maintain the defect rate at an acceptable level. For example, if the prevalence is 0.10, and the allowable defect rate is 0.05, the P_{ed} must be 0.50. This P_{ed} value of 0.50 should be considered to be a minimum value; higher P_{ed} values provide greater assurance that the maximum DR will not be exceeded. If prevalence is 0.10, and the allowable defect rate is 0.01, then the P_{ed} must be 0.90. It is worth some false rejections to maintain this level of sensitivity to errors.

Average Run Length

It must be recognized that *prevalence* is the average error rate accumulated over a long period of time. Some errors may be large and should be detected quickly. Typical causes of large errors include miscalibration and bad reagents. When these types of errors occur, their prevalence is likely to be 1.00 until they are detected and corrected. An extremely weak quality control procedure justified by Equation 8–4 could require many runs to detect a serious error. It would be unpleasant to explain to a clinician that the overall defect rate of a calcium assay is only 5%, but this 5% occurred over the 3 consecutive weeks that he was evaluating a patient for factitious hyperparathyroidism based on repeated erroneously elevated calcium results. The duration of an error before its discovery can be considered by the parameter *average run length to reject* (ARL$_r$). ARL$_r$ is the average number of runs which will occur with increased error before a run is rejected.[14] Its calculation is simple:

$$ARL_r = \frac{1}{P_{ed}},$$
Eq. 8–5

where the P$_{ed}$ is for ΔRE_c or ΔSE_c. How ARL$_r$ is interpreted is illustrated below.

Selecting a Control Procedure and Number of Replicates

Selection of control rules and numbers of replicates is always a compromise. Factors to consider include:

P$_{ed}$: As shown above, the P$_{ed}$ to detect ΔRE_c and ΔSE_c must be sufficiently high, according to Equation 8–4.

P$_{fr}$: False rejection rates of 0.01 to 0.05 are commonly accepted in the clinical laboratory. The expense of troubleshooting and repeating runs accounts for a large part of the cost of a quality control program. If ΔRE_c or ΔSE_c is low, large numbers of replicates may be required to achieve the required P$_{ed}$. If a large N is not practical, procedures involving a lower N, but higher P$_{fr}$ values may be required.

Predictive value of reject signal, PV$_r$: It is desirable to maintain the PV$_r$ as high as possible so that when rejections occur, errors can be identified and corrected. With high PV$_r$, laboratory personnel would be less inclined to habitually repeat runs until the controls are "in."

ARL$_r$: ARL$_r$ reflects the short-term performance of the control procedure.

Advantages of multirule procedures: Multirule control procedures were discussed in Chapter 4. Optimal multirule combinations for various numbers of control samples per run are summarized in Table 4–1.

Advantages of rules which can provide estimates of bias and variance for long-term quality control: It is common practice to use control rules whose limits are even multiples of the standard deviation because these rules are computationally simple and can be implemented manually. With the trend toward computerization, mean rules, range rules, and exponentially smoothed mean and chi-square rules are becoming more practical. These control rules have desirable characteristics and provide estimates of bias and imprecision.

Between-run variation: If $s_b/s_w > 1.0$, the laboratory should avoid rules whose performance characteristics are negatively affected by between-run components of variation.

Examples

The following examples from Chapter 5 demonstrate the above principles; however, it is assumed that between-run variation is negligible.

1. Design a quality control procedure for a BUN method with E_a of 4 mg/dL and 5% limits for maximum defect rate (DR = 0.05). Assume the s_t is 0.8 mg/dL, and the overall prev is 0.02.

   Critical random and systematic errors (from Equations 8–1A and 8–2A): $\Delta RE_c = 2.6s$, $\Delta SE_c = 3.4s$.

   Inherent prevalence of random error: ($E_a/s_t = 5.0$); prev (from Table 8–1) < 0.003.

   Required P_{ed} (From Equation 8–4): $P_{ed} = 0$. Since the prev < DR, low sensitivity to errors is acceptable. Two controls per run with the 1_{3s} rule will provide sufficient error detection and minimal false rejection. The rest of this example is calculated using the 1_{3s} rule with N = 2.

   Average run length (ARL_r) for an error equal to ΔRE_c: 2.4 (P_{ed} = 0.42). ARL_r for error equal to ΔSE_c: 1.1 (P_{ed} = 0.88).

   Calculated DR (Equation 8–3): 0.012 (used P_{ed} for ΔRE_c).

   Calculated PV_r (Table 4–2): 0.46 (used P_{ed} for ΔRE_c).

2. For the same BUN method as in Example 1, use 1% limits for maximum defect rate.

   Critical random and systematic errors: $\Delta RE_c = 1.9s$, $\Delta SE_c = 2.7s$.

   Inherent prevalence of random error: ($E_a/s_t = 5.0$); prev < 0.003.

   Required P_{ed}: 0.50. Acceptable performance would be provided by either the $1_{3s}/2_{2s}/R_{4s}/4_{1s}/10_x$ multirule or the $1_{2.5s}$ rule with 4 controls per run. However, the P_{fr} for the $1_{2.5s}$ rule with N = 4 is 0.05 v 0.02 for the multirule.

   ARL_r for an error equal to ΔRE_c: 1.9 (multirule, P_{ed} = 0.54). ARL_r for error equal to ΔSE_c: 1.1 (P_{ed} = 0.93).

Calculated DR: 0.01 (using P_{ed} for ΔRE_c).

PV_r: 0.36.

3. Design a quality control procedure for a calcium method with E_a = 0.5 mg/dL and 5% limits for maximum DR. Assume the s_t is 0.2 mg/dL, and the overall prev = 0.03.

   Critical random and systematic errors: ΔRE_c = 1.3s, ΔSE_c = 0.8s. Inherent prevalence of random error: $(E_a/s_t$ = 2.5); prev = 0.012. Required P_{ed}: P_{ed} = 0. Since the prev < DR, very low sensitivity to errors appears to be acceptable. Two replicates per run with the 1_{3s} rule would provide weak error detection with a very low P_{fr}. ARL_r for ΔRE_c: 20 (P_{ed} = 0.05). ARL_r for ΔSE_c: 25 (P_{ed} = 0.04). Alternatives which provide slightly improved ARL_r values are listed below:

Rule	N	P_{ed}, ΔRE_c	P_{ed}, ΔSE_c	P_{fr}	ARL_r	DR	PV_r
$1_{2.5s}$	2	0.12	0.09	0.02	11.1	0.027	0.12
$1_{2.5s}$	4	0.23	0.17	0.05	5.9	0.025	0.10
multirule	4	0.16	0.12	0.02	8.3	0.026	0.16
$\bar{X}_{0.01}/R_{0.01}$	4	0.43	0.15	0.02	6.7	0.025	0.19

4. Design a quality control procedure for a calcium method with an E_a of 0.5 mg/dL and 1% limits for the defect rate. Assume that the s_t is 0.2 mg/dL, and the overall prev is 0.02.

   Critical random and systematic errors: ΔRE_c = 0.97s, ΔSE_t = 0.17s. Inherent prevalence of random error: $(E_a/s_t$ = 2.5); prev = 0.012. The method cannot be controlled to within DR = 0.01 due to its inherent error.

5. For the same calcium method as in number 4, use 5% limits for maximum defect rate, and assume that the overall prevalence is 7%.

   Critical random and systematic errors: ΔRE_c = 1.3s, ΔSE_c = 0.8s. Inherent prevalence of random error: $(E_a/s_t$ = 2.5); prev = 0.012. Required P_{ed}: 0.28. This sensitivity to such a small increase in random error can be achieved with $R_{0.05}$ with 8 controls per run. $\bar{X}_{0.01}$ with 8 controls per run provides a P_{ed} = 0.38 for ΔSE_c. They are combined to make $\bar{X}_{0.01}/R_{0.05}$. The problem is the extremely high prevalence of error.

   ARL_r for an error equal to ΔRE_c: 3.6 (P_{ed} = 0.28). ARL_r for error equal to ΔSE_c: 2.6 (P_{ed} = 0.38).

   Calculated DR: 0.05.

   PV_r = 0.26.

EXAMPLES OF RECOMMENDED RULES

Optimal control procedures for different numbers of control replicates for general use were tabulated in Chapter 4. In these examples we consider some specific cases.

Analytical Runs With 1 Control Observation

As was stated in Chapter 4, there are certain situations for which the control results must be within the mean $\pm$ 2s limits, regardless of the repeat rate. A good example is the measurement of ethanol whenever there is likelihood that it will be used for legal purposes. If the 1_{2s} rule with N = 1 gives an adequate P_{ed}, an appropriate response to a 1_{2s} violation would be repeat testing of the control in duplicate to give a total of 3 control results. If these 3 results do not violate the combination rule $1_{3s}/(2 \text{ of } 3)_{2s}/R_{4s}$, the original rejection may be treated as a false rejection without compromising the P_{ed} of the 1_{2s} rule originally invoked.

Analytical Runs With 2 Control Observations

The use of the Westgard combination rule $1_{3s}/2_{2s}/R_{4s}/4_{1s}/10_{\bar{x}}$ for procedures with 2 control observations has been discussed in Chapter 4. The $1_{2.5s}$ rule offers approximately equal sensitivity to random and systematic errors within the first run affected by the error. The $1_{2.5s}$ rule does not reveal the type of error, and the combination rule is more sensitive to persistent systematic error in subsequent runs.

Analytical Runs With 3 Control Observations
(Blood Gases, Immunoassays)

It is common practice to use 3 control materials at different medical decision levels for blood gas analysis and immunoassays. Control at a third concentration is comforting in blood gas analysis because of its critical nature, and in immunoassays where calibration curves are nonlinear and the analytical range is very wide. Performance characteristics of a variety of control rules with 3 controls per run have been studied for blood gas analysis and immunoassay.[15-18] Optimal performance is provided by the combination rule $1_{3s}/(2 \text{ of } 3)_{2s}/R_{4s}$. Quam, Haessig, and Koch developed a comprehensive quality control program for blood gas analysis using the combination rule.[19] Eckert and Carey developed a procedure utilizing the $1_{3s}/(2 \text{ of } 3)_{2s}/R_{4s}$ rule and studied the effects of assay variables on its performance.[20] When 3 controls are included in each run, the combination rule $1_{3s}/(2$ of $3)_{2s}/R_{4s}$ is used across controls within the run, and each control is tested with the 2_{2s} rule across runs. Even when the P_{ed} for systematic error is reduced due to high between-run variation (see Chapter 6), this control procedure is the best for the detection of systematic error.

In immunoassay, the precision profile yields additional information about errors, but its performance as a control rule has not been simulated in conjunction with the recommended multirule procedures.[21]

Analytical Runs With More than 3 Controls per Run

In some situations, more than 3 control replicates are required in order to obtain an adequate P_{ed}. As seen in Example 3 above, the choice at N = 4 control replicates is between Westgard multirule $1_{3s}/2_{2s}/R_{4s}/4_{1s}/10_{\bar{x}}$ and the $\bar{X}_{.01}/R_{.01}$ combination rule. If the between-run variation is negligible, and computations required for the $\bar{X}_{.01}/R_{.01}$ rule are readily available, this combination is optimal because of its efficiency and the information it yields about the type and size of the error.

For higher numbers of control replicates per run, mean/range combinations and proportion rules perform best. For methods which produce data continuously, eg, continuous flow methods, trend analysis rules using smoothed means and standard deviations provide high P_{ed} values with a low P_{fr}, and fit well with the sequential production of control results.

Cumulative sum procedures are so affected by between-run variations that they should be avoided unless between-run variation is absent.

Multistage Control Procedures

Some automated analyzers have a definite startup cycle, which involves mixing reagents, changing reagents, calibration, etc. These automated instruments can be most effectively controlled by "nested" or "multistage"[14,22] control procedures. During the startup cycle of operation, a control procedure with a high P_{ed} is used in order to detect errors introduced by reagent or calibration changes or maintenance performed between runs. Errors are most likely to occur during startup; control procedures with a high P_{ed} are desirable. The 1_{2s} rule may be used with 2 to 4 controls for high sensitivity. If there are multiple violations, there is a high probability that an error condition really exists, and appropriate troubleshooting should be done. In effect, the control system is being asked to prove that there is no error, rather than being asked to detect an error.

For multitest analyzers, there are many opportunities for false 1_{2s} rejections. For isolated 1_{2s} rejections, rerunning controls several times is an acceptable response in order to verify that an error condition exists. The reruns and the initial control observations may be analyzed together with proportion or mean/range combination rules without sacrificing sensitivity because the number of controls will be high. When errors are detected and then remedied by reagent changes or restandardization, the method's entire startup control procedure is repeated to maintain the high P_{ed}.

Once the startup control procedures are completed successfully, it is likely that the instrument will operate in a low error prevalence mode. Low prevalence control procedures can be used, eg, the 1_{3s} rule or $1_{3.5s}$ rule with 1 or 2 controls per run. For continuous-flow instruments, single controls may be spaced to bracket patient samples; successive control results may be interpreted using the 1_{3s} rule. Trend analysis is also recommended; an additional benefit is that estimates of the mean and variance are derived.

Midway through the day, and also at the end of the day, retrospective quality control procedures using the current day's controls provide high sensitivity for detecting smaller errors, and allow correction before the next run. Mean and range or mean and chi-square rules may be used. Aronsson and Groth[23] recommended using $\overline{X}_{.01}/X^2_{.01}$ for retrospective analysis of a high-speed discrete analyzer. Carey et al studied the performance of retrospective control procedures for the IL 508 (Fisher-IL, Lexington, MA 02173) using computer simulation, and found that for 8 control observations, optimal performance was provided by the $\overline{X}_{.01}/R_{.01}$ rule using limits constructed from s_b and s_w for the $\overline{X}_{.01}$ rule (as shown in Chapter 6) and s_w for the $R_{.01}$ rule, or the combination rule $1_{3s}/(3 \text{ of } 8)_{2s}$.[24] Decision-limit cumulative sum rules suffered high P_{fr} values due to between-run variations, even though s_b/s_w was 0.85 or less for all analytes. If computerized calculation of control parameters is available, the mean/range combination is preferable because information is provided about the systematic and random error components. However, proportion rules are useful because no computation is required, and they can be quickly used for retrospective checks.

Methods with Long-Term Reagent and Calibration Stability

Instruments with stable reagents and calibration have had a dramatic impact on the operation of the clinical chemistry laboratory.

Typically, state-of-the-art analyzers initiate all of the tests requested on a sample in a random-access mode before beginning the testing of the next sample. The length of an analytical run, previously defined for batch testing, has lost its meaning and may now be considered to be as long as the time between scheduled maintenance cycles, as long as 24 hours for some analyzers.

These instruments can be controlled more easily, and with greater efficiency than previous instruments; however, specific quality control procedures must be developed for each instrument type and method after consideration of the design of the instrument and method. "Modified multistage" quality control procedures are recommended. There are 2 different requirements for "startup" control: (1) immediately after calibration of a new reagent lot, and (2) immediately after "daily" or "shift" maintenance.

The quality control procedure used after calibration of a new reagent lot should be a high prevalence control procedure, directly analogous to the multistage daily startup procedure. Four or more controls should be tested using rules like the $1_{3s}/2_{2s}/R_{4s}/4_{1s}$ combination rule when different levels of control are used, or $\bar{X}_{.01}/R_{.01}$ rules when the same control material is used. High sensitivity to shifts is required because calibration of new reagent lots is the most frequent cause of shifts on these analyzers. If a relatively large shift is apparent, immediate recalibration is suggested. If the shift appears small, the acceptability of the shift can be considered in the manner outlined in Chapter 6.

Since the performance of most state-of-the-art instruments is stable from day to day, quality control following daily or shift maintenance is considered a low-prevalence situation, analogous to the monitoring procedure above. The quality control procedure to be used following daily maintenance depends on the design of the instrument, and the operating characteristics which are affected by daily maintenance. If photometric balancing is part of daily maintenance, the control procedure should be designed to monitor the balancing. If the probe is cleaned and/or realigned, sample/reagent handling should be monitored by the startup control procedure. Whenever any reagents are prepared or reconstituted, affected tests should be controlled. Certain methods which are less stable than others may be considered high-prevalence methods; for example, ion-specific electrode methods for electrolytes. For these high-prevalence methods, the control procedure should include additional control observations.

Due to the large number of analytes measured on today's chemistry analyzers, most rejections will be false rejections. Two levels of control are usually tested for each channel, using the Westgard combination rule or the $1_{2.5s}$ rule. Violation without apparent cause should trigger repeat testing in duplicate of both controls (total N = 4); the repeat control testing is interpreted with the $1_{3s}/2_{2s}/R_{4s}/4_{1s}/10_{\bar{x}}$ combination rule or $1_{2.5s}$ rule to maintain a high P_{ed} and to avoid false acceptance. Alternatively, all 6 control results could be tested using proportion rules optimized for 6 control observations.

The frequency of maintenance and control testing may depend on the volume of testing performed on the instrument, which affects protein buildup, instrument wear, etc. Decisions about the required frequency of monitoring should not necessarily be left to the manufacturer's recommendations. Many instrument manufacturers state that controls need be run only once per day. Users of some instruments are uncomfortable with such infrequent control, and still prefer to control once per shift. The user's decision depends on his or her perception of the stability of the instrument, prevalence of error, and requirements for accreditation. Typically, controls are used liberally until enough data are available to demonstrate that instrument operation is sufficiently stable for the frequency of control to be reduced.

REFERENCES

1. Thiers RE: What are the required chemical and performance characteristics of materials used for standardization and control? In Eilers RJ, Lawson NS, Rand RN and Broughton A, eds: Quality assurance in health care: a critical appraisal of clinical chemistry. American Association for Clinical Chemistry, College of American Pathologists, Washington, DC, 1980, pp 191-206.

2. Ross JW: Control materials and calibration standards. In Werner M, ed: CRC handbook of clinical chemistry, vol. 1. CRC Press, Boca Raton, FL, 1982, pp 359-369.

3. Lawson NS, Haven GT: Analyte stability in control and reference materials. In Werner M, ed: CRC handbook of clinical chemistry, vol 1. CRC Press, Boca Raton, FL, 1982, pp 371-389.

4. Westgard JO, Klee GG: Quality assurance. In Tietz NW, ed, Textbook of clinical chemistry. Saunders, Philadelphia, 1986, pp 424-548.

5. Haven GT: Quality control in the new environment: ligand assay and TDM. Med Lab Obs, October, 1986, pp 55-58.

6. Natrella MG: Experimental statistics. National Bureau of Standards Handbook 91, U.S. Government Printing Office, Washington, DC, 1966.

7. Weisbrot IM: The statistics of quality control. In Howanitz PJ, Howanitz

JH, eds: Laboratory quality assurance. McGraw-Hill, New York, 1987, pp 20-54.

8. Burnett RW: Accurate estimation of standard deviations for quantitative methods used in clinical chemistry. Clin Chem 21:1935-1938, 1975.

9. Ross JW: Evaluation of precision. In Warner M, ed: CRC handbook of clinical chemistry, vol 1. CRC Press, Boca Raton, Florida, 1982, pp 391-422.

10. Bauer S, Kennedy JW: Applied statistics for the clinical laboratory: IV. Total imprecision. J Clin Lab Autom 2:129-133, 1982.

11. Bookbinder MJ, Panosian KJ: Correct and incorrect estimation of within-day and between-day variation. Clin Chem 32:1734-1737, 1986.

12. Bauer S, Kennedy JW: Applied statistics for the clinical laboratory: III. Variability over time. J Clin Lab Autom 2:35-40, 1982.

13. National Committee for Clinical Laboratory Standards: NCCLS tentative standard EP5-T, tentative guidelines for user evaluation of precision performance of clinical chemistry devices. Subcommittee for User Evaluation of Precision of the Evaluation Protocols Area Committee, Villanova, Pennsylvania, 1983.

14. Westgard JO, Barry PL: Cost-effective quality control: managing the quality and productivity of analytical processes. AACC Press, Washington, DC, 1986.

15. Westgard JO, Groth T: Assessment of the performance characteristics of a blood gas quality control program by use of an interactive computer simulation program. Clin Chem 26:999, 1980.

16. Schioler V: Internal quality control of immunoassays. Scan J Clin Lab Invest 44 (suppl 172):87-92, 1984.

17. Ruokonen A, Heikkila J, Leskinen E, Nyberg A, Vihko R: Internal quality control of hormone determination by RIA. Detection of clinically significant analytical errors of serum thyroxine determination. Scan J Clin Lab Invest 44 (suppl 172):93-99, 1984.

18. Carey RN, Tyvoll JL, Plaut DS, et al: Performance characteristics of some statistical quality control rules for radioimmunoassay. J Clin Immunoassay 8:245-252, 1985.

19. Quam EF, Haessig LK, Koch MJ: A comprehensive statistical quality control program for blood gas analyzers. J Med Technol 2:27-31, 1985.

20. Eckert GH, Carey RN: Application of statistical control rules to quality control in radioimmunoassay. J Clin Immunoassay 8:107-111, 1985.

21. Ekins R: The "precision profile": its use in RIA assessment and design. Ligand Q 4:33-44, 1981.

22. Westgard JO, Groth T, de Verdier C-H: Principles for developing improved quality control procedures. Scan J Clin Lab Invest 44 (suppl 172):19-41, 1984.

23. Aronsson T, Groth T: Nested control procedures for internal analytical quality control. Theoretical design and practical evaluation. Scan J Clin Lab Invest 44 (suppl 172):51-64, 1984.

24. Carey RN, Beebe S, Barry PL, Westgard JO: Assessment of performance characteristics of some quality control rules for retrospective analysis of control data from the IL 508 chemistry analyzer. Clin Chem 31:1017, 1985.

CHAPTER NINE

Quality Control in Hematology

Previous chapters have demonstrated how difficult it is to control an analytical method with a high prevalence of errors exceeding allowable error. Figure 9–1 is an actual example, from one of the authors' laboratories, which dramatically demonstrates this problem. It is a plot of the monthly tallies of repeated tests and control specimens analyzed by 3 multichannel hematology instruments for a 3 year period. There is a marked increase in the repeats and quality control specimens analyzed after July 1984, coincident with the acquisition of 3 technologically advanced multichannel hematology analyzers. These newer instruments were unable to achieve the analytical performance of their predecessors. Due to the higher frequency of large errors, considerably more quality control specimens were analyzed to confirm or rule out analytical error signaled by control rule violations. Similarly, more patient specimens were reanalyzed to either confirm the absence of significant error or to determine a more correct answer. Figure 9–1 demonstrates how much easier it is to prevent errors by using precise analytical methods with low prevalence of large errors than it is to implement procedures to detect and correct errors in poorly performing methods. *It is easier to prevent errors than to detect and correct them.*

The quality control requirements of analytical systems differ according to the methodology employed. The trend away from impedance-based hematology analyzers has just begun. Cell counting is now accomplished by impedance and laser technologies, and white cell differentiation is performed by volumetric impedance, enzyme cytochemical methods, and laser light scatter methods. These different methodologies may require not only different quality control materials but even different quality control practices.

Hematology laboratories employ a variety of quality control pro-

186

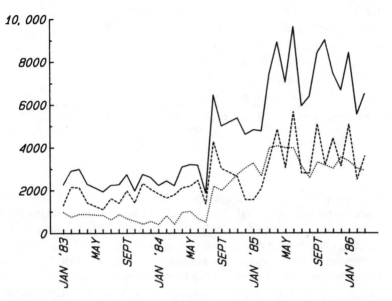

Figure 9-1 Effect of instrument selection on the monthly tally of repeated patient specimens and quality control specimens. In July 1984 all of the multichannel hematology instruments were replaced, 2 in the hematology laboratory and 1 in the Stat laboratory.

KEY: CBC–Heme ------; CBC–STAT ······; CBC–TOTAL ——.

cedures, including analysis of commercial whole blood stabilized control products, analysis of previously analyzed (retained) patient specimens, and averaging of patient data (AOP). This chapter examines the effectiveness of these control procedures and considers quality control procedures for the white cell differential and for coagulation analysis. The extent of quality control required by accrediting and regulatory agencies is also summarized.

COMMERCIAL CONTROLS

The attributes of the ideal hematology control material have been described by Bachner[1] and are listed in Table 9-1. Although control materials for clinical chemistry perform reasonably well, virtually all

Laboratory Quality Management

Table 9-1   Attributes of an ideal hematology control substance.

Inexpensive
Prolonged stability
May be sampled directly
Suspends easily and does not agglutinate
Flow characteristics similar to blood
Optical and electrical properties similar to blood
Particle size and shape similar to blood
Assayable by independent methods

Modified with permission. From Bachner P: Quality assurance in hematology. In: Howanitz PJ and Howanitz JH (eds): Laboratory quality assurance. McGraw-Hill, New York, 1987, pp 214-230.

of the commercially available hematology control products fall short of Bachner's ideal material. The period over which hematology controls are stable is quite limited, usually ranging from 30 to 60 days. Adverse shipping and storage conditions can significantly affect the stability of the control product. Each new shipment of control material requires, as a minimum, verification of the manufacturer's assayed values. Optimally, appropriate statistical control limits should be determined.

Some whole blood control materials do not simulate the behavior of patient specimens because they are composed of fixed cells or otherwise stabilized exotic components, such as avian red cells. Thus, deterioration in the analytical process may not always be detected by the commercial control. Furthermore, false rejections of the analytical run may occur, even with error-free analysis of the patient specimens, due to problems associated with the whole blood control material. As previously noted, an additional shortcoming of all types of reference sample quality control procedures is that they do not monitor the preanalytical portion of the total analytical process.

The popularity of the screening differential is spurring the development of control products which can support far more tests than ever before, 16 to 20 different parameters. This expansion, coupled with the divergent technologies for differentiating white cells, has made prolonged stability a secondary goal. The universal control product, one which can be analyzed by impedance, cytochemical, and laser-based analyzers, may become the hematologist's lodestone. Control materials optimized for one measurement technology probably will not be effective for other measurement technologies; eg, a control product designed for impedance-based white cell differentials probably will

188

not be suitable for controlling an instrument which uses cytochemical staining.

Despite these disadvantages, commercial controls have several advantages over retained patient specimens and patient data algorithms. Since they are assayed materials, they can be used to verify calibration after maintenance procedures and daily start-up. They are convenient, and are more stable than retained patient specimens.

Establishing Control Ranges

Before hematology control products are shipped, their manufacturer assays them on a variety of instruments. Expected ranges are derived from these studies and are documented in the control product package insert. These ranges should not be used for run acceptance decisions as they are too broad for effective quality control. To illustrate this point, a commercial control material's expected ranges can be transformed into z-scores of a given laboratory's standard deviation from the mean. This transformation is performed by dividing the maximum allowable deviation by the laboratory's usual standard deviation for that particular control material. This quantity is the maximal allowable excursion (in standard deviations) which can occur before an error condition is signaled. Thus, if a package insert documents the maximum allowable deviation for hemoglobin to be 0.3 g/dL at a mean of 12 g/dL and the standard deviation of the assay is 0.1 g/dL at a level of 12 g/dL, the allowable excursion is 0.3/0.1, or 3 standard deviations.

Most hematology control manufacturer's allowable excursions are at least 3 standard deviations from the mean. A quality control procedure which uses error limits of 3 standard deviations is equivalent to using the 1_{3s} control rule. Use of the 1_{3s} control rule alone with only 2 or 3 control replicates yields very low error detection. Wide control limits are provided by the control manufacturer to allow for between-instrument and between-laboratory variation.

Use of manufacturer-supplied control limits thwarts the application of statistical quality control. If statistical quality control is to be used effectively, laboratory- and instrument-specific control ranges must be determined. These control limits should be obtained before the control material is placed into service. During this "break-in period," the time interval after the new control material is received and before the old control material expires, the new control material should be analyzed twice daily for a minimum of 5 days, preferably for 10 days, so the target mean of the control observations can be accurately estimated.

The analysis of the control material should be spread over as many days as possible to prevent short-term systematic error from biasing the mean. The standard deviation of these 10 to 20 observations will be lower than the long-term standard deviation because it is obtained over a short time compared to the lifetime of the control material. It should not be used to calculate the control limits. Rather, the control limits should be derived from this mean and the accepted long-term within-instrument standard deviation, s_{lt}. For example, in the normal range, a typical s_{lt} for hemoglobin measured by the S + IV is 0.10 to 0.12 g/dL; for red blood count it is 0.05×10^{12}/L.[2]

Although the manufacturer-supplied mean and range should not be used for run acceptance decisions, they do have useful functions. If they have been determined accurately, they provide benchmarks for assessing a hematology analyzer's overall systematic and random errors.

Multirule Control Procedure

In hematology, it is reasonable to consider 3 control observations at once, since 3 different control levels are typically assayed at least once daily: low, normal, and elevated. In Chapters 4 and 8, combination rules using the $(2 \text{ of } 3)_{2s}$ and R_{4s} rules were recommended for situations with 3 control replicates. The $(2 \text{ of } 3)_{2s}$ control rule is violated if any 2 of the last 3 control observations are beyond the same mean $\pm$ 2s limit. The R_{4s} control rule is violated if any 2 of the last 3 control observations exceed opposite mean $\pm$ 2s limits. Figure 9–2 diagrams how the $(2 \text{ of } 3)_{2s}$ and R_{4s} control rules can be violated. If the $(2 \text{ of } 3)_{2s}$ rule is violated, systematic error is more likely. If the R_{4s} rule is violated, random error is more probable.

If the 1_{3s} control rule is added to the $(2 \text{ of } 3)_{2s}/R_{4s}$ combination rule, the sensitivity to random and systematic error is increased without significant increases in the P_{fr}. Figure 9–3 shows the power functions for the $1_{3s}/(2 \text{ of } 3)_{2s}/R_{4s}$ control procedure. The probability of false rejection for this combination is 2% for 3 control observations; it increases to approximately 5% for 9 control observations. Not all of the tests produced by a multichannel hematology analyzer need to be monitored with the $1_{3s}/(2 \text{ of } 3)_{2s}/R_{4s}$ control procedure, however. We suggest that only those tests which are directly measured and must be controlled as tightly as possible should be monitored, eg, hemoglobin (Hgb) and red blood cell count (RBC). Calculated results, such as red cell distribution width, mean corpuscular hemoglobin (MCH), and mean corpuscular hemoglobin concentration (MCHC), may better be controlled with control rules like the 1_{3s} rule which has a lower P_{fr}.

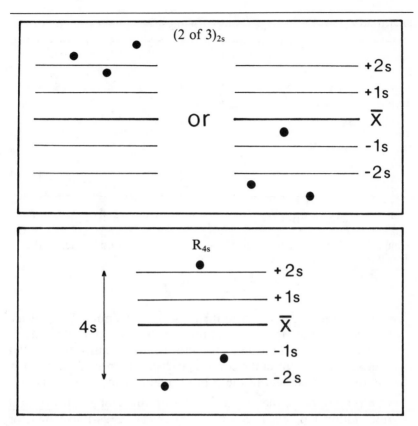

Figure 9–2 Examples of violations of the (2 of 3)$_{2s}$ and R$_{4s}$ control rules.

This approach is statistically valid since these results are not independent, but depend on the values obtained for the tests which are measured directly.

Figure 9–4 shows how the 1$_{3s}$/(2 of 3)$_{2s}$/R$_{4s}$ control procedure can be implemented in the hematology laboratory. If all 3 control materials are analyzed, the following protocol can be employed for the directly measured parameters:

The control results are screened by comparing them to their mean ± 2s limits. If the results are within their mean ± 2s limits, the instrument is judged to be in control, and the patient specimens can be analyzed without further checking of control results.

If any control result exceeds the mean ± 2s limits, the control

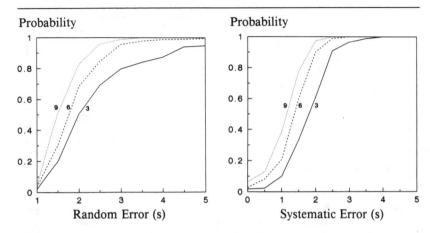

Figure 9–3 Power functions for the $1_{3s}/(2\ of\ 3)_{2s}/R_{4s}$ control rule for the detection of systematic and random errors.

results are then compared to their mean ± 3s limits; if any of the results exceed the mean ± 3s limits, there is a high probability of analytical error and the analytical process must be investigated. (Of course, if a problem in the control product is suspected, then a new aliquot or a specimen of the control product should be analyzed).

Control results are then investigated with the $(2\ of\ 3)_{2s}/R_{4s}$ control rule, within the run. If a test exceeds mean ± 2s limits on 2 or more control materials, the type of error must be determined (systematic v random) and the analytical process investigated.

If a test exceeds mean ± 2s limits on only 1 control result, the previous result for that material is investigated to determine whether a 2_{2s} violation has occurred. The 2_{2s} rule is used instead of the $(2\ of\ 3)_{2s}$ rule to reduce false rejections.

After a $1_{3s}/(2\ of\ 3)_{2s}/R_{4s}$ combination rule violation has been investigated and appropriate measures have been followed, the controls should be retested in duplicate to obtain 6 observations. This ensures adequate P_{ed} for random error and still maintains an acceptable P_{fr}.

The above procedure may be used with any combination of control materials and replicates which yields 3 control results (whether 3 different control materials are utilized or the same material is analyzed 3 times).

192

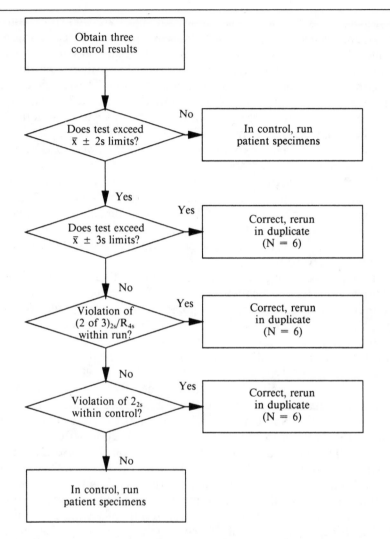

Figure 9-4   Implementation of the $1_{3s}/(2 \text{ of } 3)_{2s}/R_{4s}$ control procedure.

RETAINED PATIENT SPECIMENS

Many protocols employing retained specimens have been recommended for the quality control of hematology analyzers. Retained specimens are those which have been previously analyzed when the instrument has been in a state of control, as indicated by the results of

193

commercial control analysis. These specimens are then refrigerated and reanalyzed at a later time, with the new values compared to original values. Significant variation between the original and current values indicates one of three phenomena: significant change in the instrument, specimen interchange, or specimen deterioration. The last case, that of specimen deterioration, should be infrequent as EDTA anticoagulated blood specimens are stable for up to 24 hours when refrigerated.[3]

The protocols which use retained specimens vary greatly.[4] One protocol requires that approximately 5% of the total workload be reanalyzed.[5] Another protocol specifies that the difference between original and duplicate measurements be plotted daily,[6] while another requires that the average difference of 5 retained specimens be used.[7] Other protocols use the calculation of the standard deviation of duplicate measurements, while still another uses a target mean value derived from 5 initial replicate measurements with reanalysis of the control specimen every 10 to 15 specimens.[8]

Cembrowski et al studied the effectiveness of various control procedures using retained patient specimens.[4] They found that the variation of the red cell parameters (Hgb, RBC, mean corpuscular volume [MCV], MCH, MCHC, and hematocrit [Hct]) of patient specimens retained and analyzed over a 40 hour period on a Coulter S+IV was equivalent to the variation of a Coulter commercial control product analyzed over 30 days. Control limits for the red cell parameters of retained patient specimens can thus be derived from the long-term standard deviations of commercial controls. They found more variation in the white blood cell (WBC) count and the platelet count and suggested wider control limits, $\pm$ 0.75 $\times$ 10^9/L for WBC and $\pm$ 30 $\times$ 10^9/L for platelet counts. Computer simulation of the use of retained patient specimens on the Coulter S+IV demonstrated that the $(2 \text{ of } 3)_{2s}$ control rule is the most effective control rule based on the performance characteristics and the small number of retained specimens which should be reanalyzed. For interpreting results of testing on retained patient specimens, the $(2 \text{ of } 3)_{2s}$ condition occurs whenever the differences between the current results and the original results for a parameter exceed $\pm$ 2s for 2 of the 3 retained patient specimens. It is important to note that the differences are not between the current result and the mean, but between the current result and the original result. The rule is invoked whenever the absolute difference exceeds 2s; it may be either positive or negative.

Power functions for the $(2 \text{ of } 3)_{2s}$ rule applied to retained patient specimens are shown in Figures 9–5 and 9–6. Figure 9–5 shows that the capabilities of this procedure to detect systematic error are reduced

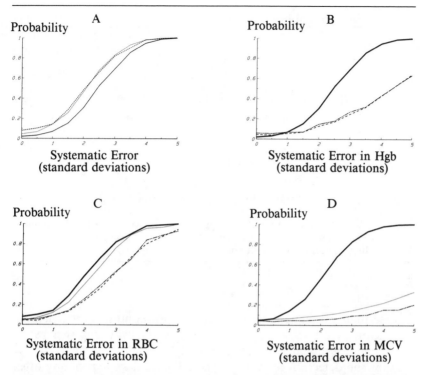

Figure 9–5 Power function curves for the detection of systematic error for retained patient specimens using the $(2 \text{ of } 3)_{2s}$ control rule. Figure 9–5 A compares the power function curves for the detection of systematic error in Hgb, RBC, and MCV when differences between replicate Hgb, RBC, and MCV values, respectively, are evaluated. In Figures 9–5: B–D, systematic error is applied in either Hgb, RBC, or MCV with power function curves presented for the measured and calculated parameters.

when the derived quantities Hct, MCH, and MCHC are monitored. Thus, it is recommended that only the directly measured parameters, ie, Hgb, RBC, MCV, platelets, and WBC, be monitored with this procedure. Figures 9–5 and 9–6 also demonstrate that this procedure is more sensitive to systematic error than to random error.

The performance of multirule control procedures applied to control data will always be superior to the $(2 \text{ of } 3)_{2s}$ rule applied to retained patient specimens. The basis for the evaluation of control data is the control mean, which is precisely known. The basis for the evaluation of retained patient specimen data is the first result, which is no more

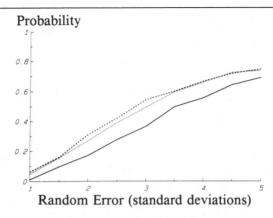

Figure 9–6   Power function curves of the $(2 \text{ of } 3)_{2s}$ control rules for the detection of random error when differences between replicate Hgb, RBC, and MCV values of retained patient specimens are evaluated.

KEY: Hgb ———; RBC ------; MCV ⋯⋯.

precise than subsequent results. Control procedures for retained patient samples are thus inherently less powerful with any increase in P_{ed} being accompanied by an increased P_{fr}. The P_{fr} of the $(2 \text{ of } 3)_{2s}$ rule for the detection of RBC errors is higher than that of any other directly measured parameter; P_{ed} is also higher. Use of a less sensitive retained patients procedure, eg, the $(2 \text{ of } 3)_{2.5s}$ rule for RBC would be appropriate in a quality control system which also uses Bull's algorithm, because of the algorithm's high sensitivity to RBC errors (see below). The $(2 \text{ of } 3)_{2.5s}$ rule would also have a more acceptable P_{fr}.

Cembrowski et al recommend that 3 normal range patient specimens be retained after initial analysis and then be reanalyzed at regular intervals; for example, every 8 hours. After each reanalysis, differences between the initial and the replicate determinations should be calculated and compared to the ± 2s limits. If the differences between the initial and replicate determinations exceed 2s for 2 of the 3 specimens, an out-of-control situation exists. This retained specimen quality control procedure assumes that normal range specimens are reanalyzed. The standard deviation of most analytical methods is proportional to concentration. Use of specimens which are significantly higher in concentration will result in a higher than expected P_{fr}. Similarly, use of low-level specimens will result in a lower P_{ed}.

USE OF PATIENT DATA ALGORITHMS—
MOVING AVERAGES

The capability of control procedures which employ averages of patient data (AOP) to detect systematic error was demonstrated in Chapter 7. The performance of any AOP control procedure depends on specific characteristics of the patient data and the control procedure. In order of decreasing importance, these characteristics are: (1) the ratio of the standard deviation of the patient population (s_p) to the standard deviation of the analytic method (s_a); (2) the number of patient results averaged (N); (3) the control limits and thus the probability of false rejection; (4) the truncation limits for exclusion of patient data to be averaged; and (5) the population lying outside the truncation limits.

The most important parameters, s_p/s_a and N, are closely related. The number of test results which must be averaged to efficiently detect systematic error varies with the ratio s_p/s_a. For large ratios, very large numbers of patient values must be averaged; for ratios approaching 1, comparatively few patient results must be averaged to obtain the same information about systematic error. Table 9–2 illustrates this relationship, showing the number of patient values which must be averaged to obtain a 50% probability of detecting a 2 standard deviation shift in the analytical method.

Of the directly measured parameters, platelet averages demonstrate the greatest utility for indicating the presence of systematic error. After exclusion of outlying platelet populations, 70 patient platelet results must be averaged to efficiently detect a 2s shift in the platelet count. Considerably more patient values of the other directly measured parameters would have to be averaged to provide meaningful information about the existence of systematic error. However, relatively few MCHC and MCH values need to be averaged to detect systematic error. This explains why Dorsey[9] and Bull et al[10] found the averages of patient indices useful for the quality control of hematology analyzers.

Bull and associates recommended an averaging technique (now commonly known as "Bull's algorithm") which uses the average of groups of 20 consecutive patient red blood cell indices. An average outside its control limits would require investigation and appropriate action. The advantages of such an algorithm over commercial control material include economy and the frequent monitoring of analytical performance.[11] Bull's algorithm has now been implemented by vir-

Table 9-2 Comparison of s_p/s_a and the number of patient values required to detect a $2s_a$ shift in a Coulter S+IV with a probability of 50%.

Test	s_p/s_a	N
MCHC	1.7	<20
Platelets	6	70
MCH	7	100
MCV	11	250
WBC	12	300
Hct	16	400
RBC	16	400
Hgb	23	800

Note: The control limits for the mean are set as 99% confidence limits: Mean $\pm$ 2.58 $s_a/\sqrt{N}$. Values of s_p were derived from the standard deviation of patient test results with outlying populations excluded. Values of s_a were obtained from the standard deviation of a midlevel control analyzed by a Coulter S+IV over a 1 month period.

tually all manufacturers of multiparameter hematology analyzers. The formula for the averaging technique follows:

$$\overline{X}_{B,i} = \overline{X}_{B,i-1} + \text{sgn}\left[\sum_{j=1}^{N} \text{sgn}\,(X_{j,i} - \overline{X}_{B,i-1})\sqrt{|X_{j,i} - \overline{X}_{B,i-1}|}\right]$$
$$\times \frac{\left[\sum_{j=1}^{N} \text{sgn}\,(X_{j,i} - \overline{X}_{B,i-1})\sqrt{|X_{j,i} - \overline{X}_{B,i-1}|}\right]^2}{N}.$$

In the formula, the symbol "sgn" denotes the operation that returns $+1$ if the sign of the following bracketed formula is positive, or -1 if the sign of the formula is negative. $\overline{X}_{B,i}$ denotes the new Bull's mean, $\overline{X}_{B,i-1}$ denotes the last Bull's mean. While the formula is complex, the principle of Bull's algorithm is simple. The individual steps in the algorithm as applied to MCV are outlined in Table 9-3. For each batch of 20 patient specimen results, the differences between each of the patient indices (MCH or MCHC or MCV) and the last Bull's mean are calculated. The square root of each of these 20 differences is then calculated with the sign of the individual differences affixed to the square roots. Thus if a trend results in many MCVs which are less than the previous Bull's mean, many of the differences and the square roots of the differences will be less than 0. The square roots of the differences are then summed and divided by 20. The resulting term

Table 9-3   Steps in calculation of Bull's mean ($\bar{X}_b$).

1. Get new batch of 20 indices, eg, MCVs.
2. Calculate differences between X_B and all MCVs.
3. Calculate square roots of differences, preserving sign.
4. Sum square roots, preserving sign.
5. Square sum of square roots, preserving sign.
6. Divide by 20 to get average difference.
7. Add to X_B to get new X_B.

can be considered the square root of the average deviation from the last Bull's mean. To make this term an average deviation, it is then squared with its sign preserved. This average deviation of the current batch is added to the current Bull's mean to produce the new Bull's mean. The square root function "trims" the data, reducing the effects of outliers, and the incorporation of the average deviation into Bull's mean "smooths" the data, lessening the effects of random errors and abnormal patient results.

Two different control procedures are used to evaluate Bull's mean. The most popular control procedure compares Bull's mean to control limits defined as $(1 \pm 0.03) \times$ the stable mean index.[10] In other words, if Bull's mean is more than 3% from its usual value, either an analytical problem exists or else the patient population has changed enough to cause shift in the patient indices. Another control procedure, called Bull's multirule algorithm, requires 1 of 2 conditions to be satisfied: either Bull's mean of 1 of the red blood cell indices is outside its 3% limits or the average of the last 3 Bull's means is outside its 2% limits.[12] Graphical presentation of the patient indices expedites trend detection and correction. Figure 9-7 illustrates control charts for mean patient indices during the malfunction and correction of the Coulter S+IV. Both the 2% and 3% limits have been drawn.

The stable patient mean indices are determined by collecting at least 500 to 1000 sets of MCH, MCV, and MCHC values over a period of at least a month during the problem-free operation of the hematology analyzer. The indices are then averaged. Collecting fewer than 500 sets of indices can result in an inaccurate mean index; similarly, collecting data over a short period increases the chance of biased indices, due either to sampling patients with aberrant indices or not sampling from enough runs to allow between-run variances to "average out."

Koepke and Protextor have reported on their 4 years' experience

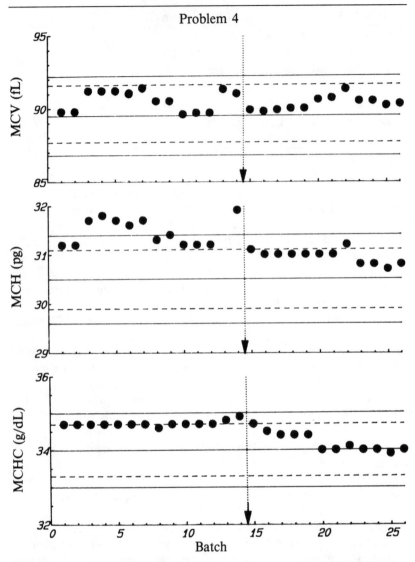

Figure 9-7   Control charts for Bull's algorithm, with 2% and 3% limits. The effect of an error in red blood cell count on the mean patient indices is shown. A solenoid had not been functioning properly over a period of several days, but was not discovered until RBC counts were affected. Malfunction of the solenoid resulted in the bubbles in the RBC bath being unable to enter the system properly. A new solenoid was installed at batch 14 and the MCH and MCHC normalized.

(Data courtesy of M. Wilson)

using Bull's algorithm and 3% control limits in lieu of commercial controls, which were discontinued during the study.[13] Forty-two significant instrument malfunctions were detected. The MCHC was affected in 83% of the malfunctions, the MCH in 60%, and the MCV in 36%.

Cembrowski and Westgard evaluated Bull's algorithm using computer simulation studies.[14] Varying amounts of systematic error, expressed as multiples of the long-term standard deviation, were introduced into simulated patient data for hemoglobin, red blood cell count, or mean corpuscular volume. The resulting indices were averaged in groups of 20 using Bull's algorithm. The number of batches with indices outside of the 3% limits was tabulated and power function graphs were generated. Figure 9–8 shows the power functions for detecting error in hemoglobin and RBC (monitored by the average MCH and MCHC) and MCV (monitored by the average MCV and MCHC). Figure 9–8A shows that Bull's mean can detect a 3s shift in hemoglobin only about 2% of the time after a single batch of 20 MCHs is averaged. The probability of error detection after 5 batches (100 patient values) of MCHs have been averaged is about 17%. Figure 9–8B shows that the probability of detecting a 3s error in hemoglobin using the average MCHC is low even with many batches. The probability of detecting error in the RBC is shown in Figures 9–8C and D. Detection of 3s errors is about 70% when the MCHC is averaged, even after only 1 batch. The averaged MCH and MCHC are both capable of detecting 3s shifts in RBC about 80% of the time after 9 batches. Figures 9–8E and 9–8F show that only large shifts in the MCV can be detected when averaging the MCV or the MCHC.

Cembrowski and Westgard also demonstrated that the inclusion of populations with outlying values, such as neonates and oncology patients, changes the performance characteristics of the system. Usually, there is decreased detection of certain kinds of errors and increased probability of false rejection. They recommended caution in discontinuing the use of control materials.

Lunetzky and Cembrowski used computer simulations to evaluate the performance of the Bull multirule control procedure,[12] in which a test is considered to be out of control if either its Bull's average is outside of its 3% limits, or the average of its last 3 Bull's averages is outside of its 2% limits.[15] Figure 9–9 shows power function curves for Bull's multirule and, for comparison, the power function curve of the single rule procedure for the ninth batch of simulated patient data. The multirule procedure is more sensitive to error than the single rule procedure. In particular, the detection of 2s to 3s shifts in hemoglobin

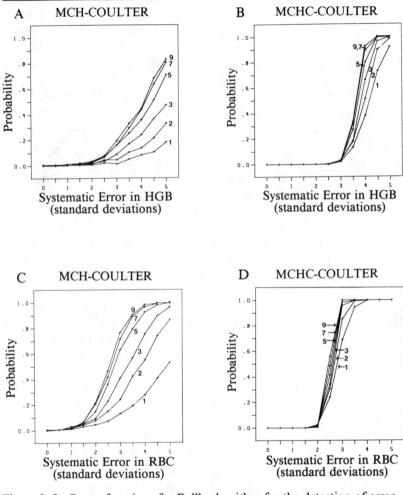

Figure 9–8 Power functions for Bull's algorithm for the detection of error in hemoglobin (A, B), red cell count (C, D) and MCV (E, F). The probability of rejection is plotted against the size of the systematic error (SE) expressed in multiples of the longterm standard deviation (S). The numbers 1, 3, 5, 7, and 9 correspond to the number of batches of 20 patient specimens analyzed. Three graphs are needed to show the effects of analytical error on MCHC, because MCHC is derived from Hgb, RBC, and MCV. Only 2 graphs are needed for MCH (derived from Hgb and RBC) and only 1 graph for MCV (directly measured).

Reproduced with permission. From Cembrowski GS, Westgard, JO: Quality control of multichannel hematology analyzers: evaluation of Bull's algorithm. Am J Clin Pathol 83:337-345, 1985.

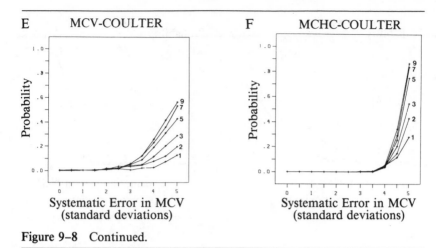

Figure 9–8   Continued.

and 3s to 4s shifts in MCV is much improved. Detection of RBC shifts is dramatically improved, with 2s shifts being readily detected. In fact, this level of error detection in the RBC may not be desirable, since it is neither analytically nor clinically significant. The magnitude of error detected in hemoglobin or the MCV is significant and should be corrected. Table 9–4 compares the minimum error detected 50% of the time by the single-rule and the multirule procedures.

The Bull's simulation results are strictly applicable to the Coulter S+IV. These results are not valid for hematology analyzers which require frequent recalibration. They are also not valid for instruments which produce indices that have a larger s_p than that provided by the Coulter S+IV. For example, s_p for MCHC on the Technicon H1 is on the order of 1.7 compared to 0.6 g/dL on the Coulter.[16] The power of MCHC to detect errors is reduced in comparison to the Coulter. With such an instrument, it may be wiser to increase the number of patient specimens averaged in a batch (eg, to 30 or 40) or to increase the frequency of testing of commercial controls and retained patient specimens.

A balanced use of control materials, moving averages, and retained patient specimen testing is advised.[2] All 3 control procedures can detect systematic error. Generally, the sensitivity of Bull's multirule algorithm to systematic error is equivalent to a multirule control procedure using stabilized control materials. A minimum of 3 batches, however (60 specimens) must be averaged with Bull's algorithm to yield a 50% probability of detecting a 3s shift. Although random errors may be

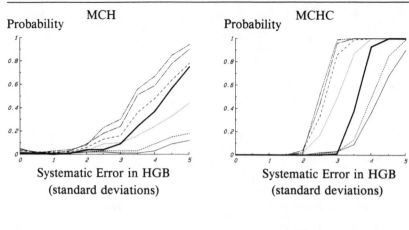

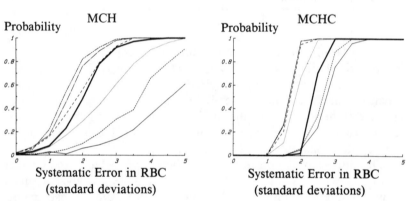

Figure 9–9 The power function curves of the multirule procedure for the detection of systematic error in Hgb, RBC, and MCV. The probability of rejection is plotted versus the size of analytic shift expressed in multiples of the long term standard deviation. The curves are labeled with the number of batches of 20 patient specimens analyzed. The bold line represents the performance of the single rule procedure for the ninth batch of patient specimens. Three graphs are needed to show the effects of analytical error on MCHC, because MCHC is derived from Hgb, RBC and MCV. Only 2 graphs are needed for MCH (derived from Hgb and RBC) and only 1 graph for MCV (directly measured).

From Lunetzky ES, Cembrowski GS: Performance characteristics of Bull's multirule algorithm for the quality control of multichannel hematology analyzers. Am J Clin Pathol 88:634-638, 1987.

KEY: N=1 ——; N=2 ---; N=3 ·····; N=5 ————; N=7 –·–·–; N=9 –··—··; N=9 (3% Limits) ——.

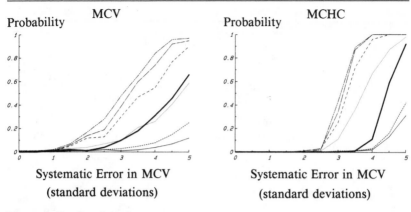

Figure 9-9 Continued.

KEY: N=1 ——; N=2 ---; N=3 ····; N=5 ----; N=7 -·-·-; N=9 —··—··; N=9 (3% Limits) ——.

detected by retained patient specimen procedures, control material procedures are more sensitive to random error. Control materials can be analyzed at any time without the requirement to accumulate patient specimen results, and thus are especially useful at instrument startup and after maintenance and recalibration. Perhaps the greatest value of moving averages and retained patient specimen procedures is that they do permit control of the multichannel analyzer during the intervals when control materials are not being run. The combination of startup quality control with control materials and continuing control with moving patient averages and retained patient specimens is an example of multistage quality control.

WHITE CELL DIFFERENTIAL COUNTS

The imprecision and inaccuracy of the routine manual differential count have been well documented.[17-21] The imprecision is attributable to nonrandom cell distribution on the wedge smear, cell identification errors, and statistical sampling error due to the small (100 to 200 cells) sample size.[22] These factors also contribute to inaccuracy, as does the lack of agreement on standardized morphological definitions of certain cell types, most notably band neutrophils.[23] Thus, if the goal of the manual differential count is a precise and accurate enumeration of blood cell types, both accuracy and precision are poor unless very large numbers of cells are examined. Bull has argued that a better statement

Table 9–4 Comparison of sensitivity to systematic error for single-rule and multirule Bull's algorithms.

		Minimum Error Detected 50% of the time (9 batches averaged)	
		Control Procedure	
Analyte	Averaged Parameter	Single rule	Multirule
Hgb,	MCH	$4.2s_a$	$3.2s_a$
$s_a = 0.1g/dL$	MCHC	$3.5s_a$	$2.3s_a$
(CV = 0.8%)			
RBC,	MCH	$2.0s_a$	$1.2s_a$
$s_a = 0.05 \times 10^{12}/L$	MCHC	$2.2s_a$	$1.5s_a$
(CV = 1.3%)			
MCV,	MCV	$4.5s_a$	$3.0s_a$
$s_a = 0.60fL$	MCHC	$4.3s_a$	$3.0s_a$
(CV = 0.7%)			

Abbreviations: CV = coefficient of variation.

Reproduced with permission. From Lunetzky ES, Cembrowski GS: Performance characteristics of Bull's multirule algorithm for the quality control of multichannel hematology analyzers. Am J Clin Pathol 88:634-638, 1987.

of purpose for the manual differential count is that "a qualified observer has examined the blood film for a broad spectrum of abnormalities."[24] He proposes a quality control program centered around "expert morphology review," the review of all blood smears showing significant abnormalities by a highly competent morphologist. He also suggests the use of the laboratory computer to track the frequency with which certain cell types are identified by each technologist, comparing that frequency to the laboratory mean. Other intriguing suggestions are made, and the interested reader is referred to Bull's excellent discussion.[24]

A simplified approach would be to periodically submit to each technologist carefully chosen blood smears containing small numbers of abnormal cells. The technologists would be asked to "screen" the slides rather than do a formal differential count. The ability of a technologist to detect these low-frequency abnormalities would establish him or her as a "qualified observer." In order to guarantee specificity, normal peripheral smears should be included in this program. This approach can be used along with expert morphology review to provide a comprehensive quality control program for the manual differential count.

Regardless of the vigor with which the manual differential count is pursued, there is a large statistical sampling error involved, which can only be reduced by greatly increasing the number of cells counted.[23] The automated screening differential instruments afford the opportunity to count numbers of cells in the thousands, thus greatly reducing the statistical sampling error and allowing for a high degree of precision. The quality control of the automated screening differential count offers a new challenge to the laboratorian. For example, it has been recently demonstrated that using the absolute numbers of cells as the controlled parameter is more sensitive to systematic error than white cell percentages.[25] Clearly, the imprecision of manual counts (with limited numbers of cells counted) prevents their being used as a trustworthy control procedure for the automated screening differential.

COAGULATION

Multirule quality control procedures are applicable in coagulation analyses. Cembrowski and Patrick studied the performance of a multirule procedure to control automated prothrombin time (PT) and activated partial thromboplastin time (aPTT) analyses using 3 control materials,[26] and found that the 4_{1s} and 10_x rules were overly sensitive to small, clinically unimportant shifts. Thus, the 1_{2s} control rule was used for screening subsequent control results, and violations of only the 1_{3s}, 2_{2s}, and R_{4s} rules required rejection of a run.

PT and aPTT control results were monitored using a multirule chart, similar to that shown in Figure 9-10, which tabulates results from several control materials according to the distance from their respective means. The chart serves as both a numeric tabulation and a graphical chart, and enables the evaluation of control data across and within control materials simultaneously. Although it is demonstrated for coagulation quality control, it is broadly applicable.

Duplicate testing of the PT and aPTT is commonly practiced. Hagemann, Lunetzky, and Cembrowski used computer simulation of patient data to first optimize and then evaluate the error detection capabilities of duplicate PT and aPTT testing.[27] A maximum allowable difference of 3% between duplicates yielded an optimal error detection rate for the PT. For the aPTT, the optimal maximum allowable difference was 6%. However, the power functions demonstrate that, even at these optimized limits, the probability of detecting large random errors is only moderate. In addition, the probability of falsely accepting

```
 5/22/85                                                                 4W099   4W090
                                          APTT                           4R442   4W472
                                                                                 4W475
    LEVEL  I      52.7   56.2   59.7    63.2      66.7   70.2   73.7
    LEVEL  II     70.0   75.0   80.0    85.0      90.0   95.0  100.0
    VER. NORM     27.8   28.8   29.8    30.8      31.8   32.8   33.8
                   ↓      ↓      ↓       ↓         ↓      ↓      ↓
  I DATE I  TIME  I      I -3s II -2s I -1s I MEAN I +1s I +2s II +3s I      I INIT I COMMENTS    I
  I 8/25 I  1 PM  I      I     II     I     I      I 65.5 I    II     I      I CLR  I             I
  I      I        I      I     II     I     I      I 89.3 I    II     I      I      I             I
  I      I        I      I     II     I     I      I 30.9 I    II     I      I      I             I
  I      I  4 PM  I      I     II     I     I      I 31.4 I    II     I      I      I             I
  I      I  5 PM  I      I     II 29.6 I    I      I      I    II     I      I MM   I             I
  I      I        I      I     II     I 61.7 I     I      I    II     I      I      I             I
  I      I        I      I     II     I 80.6 I     I      I    II     I      I      I             I
  I      I  7 PM  I      I     II     I     I      I 31.3 I    II     I      I MM   I             I
  I      I  9 PM  I      I     II 29.6 I    I      I      I    II     I      I RON  I             I
  I      I        I      I     II 58.7 I    I      I      I    II     I      I      I             I
  I      I        I      I     II 77.2 I    I      I      I    II     I      I      I             I
  I      I 11 PM  I      I     II     I     I      I      I 32.6 II    I      I MM   I             I
  I 8/26 I12:30 AMI      I     II     I 30.3 I     I      I    II     I      I CLR  I             I
  I      I        I      I     II 78.0 I    I      I      I    II     I      I      I             I
  I      I        I      I     II 59.6 I    I      I      I    II     I      I      I             I
  I      I  2:30  I      I     II     I     I      I 31.1 I    II     I      I      I             I
  I      I  4:30  I      I     II     I     I      I      I 32.1 II    I      I      I             I
  I      I        I      I     II     I     I      I 66.2 I    II     I      I      I             I
  I      I        I      I     II     I     I      I 88.7 I    II     I      I      I             I
  I      I  6:30  I      I     II     I     I      I      I 32.7 II    I      I      I             I
  I      I 10 AM  I      I     II 29.4 I    I      I      I    II     I      I JL   I             I
  I      I        I      I     II     I 80.3 I     I      I    II     I      I      I             I
  I      I        I      I     II     I 61.2 I     I      I    II     I      I      I             I
  I      I 12:30  I      I     II 30.1 I    I      I      I    II     I      I      I             I
  I      I        I      I     II     I     I      I 63.6 I    II     I      I      I             I
```

Figure 9-10 Example of a multirule control chart for aPTT analyses. The mean, mean ± 1s, mean ± 2s and mean ± 3s limits are printed at the top of the control chart for the three control levels. The mean ± 2s limits are represented by the double vertical lines.

duplicates with significant error, and the probability of rejecting duplicates without significant error is considerable. Thus, routine duplicate PT and aPTT analysis can be discontinued because of its poor performance as a quality control procedure and because of the excellent analytical precision of today's coagulation analyzers.

ACCREDITING AND REGULATORY AGENCY REQUIREMENTS

While guidelines for quality control practices in the hematology laboratory have been published by various organizations, they should be considered as minimal guidelines. Supplementary quality control procedures can thus be developed and implemented.

The Joint Commission on Accreditation of Healthcare Organizations (JCAHO) requirements for hematology are vague as to the control materials to be tested and their frequency of testing.[28] They specify that: "Each instrument or other device is calibrated/tested, as appropriate, on each day of use. . . . Reference materials and methods are tested on each day of use against known standards or controls within the range of clinically significant values . . . standard deviation, coef-

Table 9–5 Summary of HSQB interpretive guidelines for hematology.

Test Procedure	Number of Controls and Frequency	Type of Control
Manual hemoglobin	2 levels/8 hours	2AC or 2S or 1AC and 1 RS or 1S and 1RS
Manual hematocrit	1 level/8 hours	AC or RS
Manual RBC	1 level/8 hours	AC or procedural control
Manual WBC	1 level/8 hours	AC or procedural control
Manual platelets	1 level/8 hours	AC or procedural control
Automated multichannel hematology analyzer	2 levels/8 hours	2AC or 1AC and 1RS or 2RS
Prothrombin time	2 levels/8 hours and with new vials of thromboplastin	2AC
Partial thromboplastin time	2 levels/8 hours	2AC

Abbreviations: AC = assayed control(s).
S = standard(s).
RS = patient specimen(s) previously analyzed in same run as assayed control.
Procedural control. A procedural control for RBC, WBC, or platelet counts involves duplicate analysis by 1 or 2 individuals and comparison of differences of duplicates to acceptable limits. Platelet counts and WBC may also be compared to the blood smear estimate.

From Interpretive Guidelines for Independent Laboratories, Revision 189, C-78.27, 06-86 and Revision 170, C-79, 12-84. Health Care Financing Administration, United States Government, 1986.

ficient of variation, or other statistical estimates of precision are determined by random replicate testing of specimens ... The accuracy and precision of blood cell counts and hematocrit and hemoglobin measurements are tested on each day of use. ... Tests such as the one-stage prothrombin time are run in duplicate, unless the laboratory can demonstrate that low frequency of random error, or high precision, make this unnecessary."

The College of American Pathologists (CAP) in the Checklist for Hematology Laboratory Accreditation specifies that "an appropriate number of analyses of stabilized control or previously analyzed patient specimens" be performed each shift.[29] No interpretive control limits are proposed. If moving averages of red cell indices are used, the CAP specifies that: (a) control limits for red cell drift be "appropriately sensitive;" (b) white cell and platelet controls be analyzed on each shift

209

of use; (c) at least 2 previously analyzed patient specimens or stabilized control material samples be analyzed each shift; (d) the control procedure be "well defined and appropriately sensitive to drift in analyzer calibration." If an automated differential counter is used, there must be "periodic evaluation of its performance using defined limits of agreement with manually counted control slides or a stabilized control material containing at least 2 classes of white cell surrogate particles." As for prothrombin time (PT) and activated partial thromboplastin time (aPTT), CAP requires that ". . . the automated system [be] checked each shift with controls or against a manual procedure."

The hematology guidelines of the Health Standards and Quality Bureau (HSQB) of the Health Care Financing Administration (HCFA[30]) are summarized in Table 9-5. The HSQB permits various combinations of assayed stabilized controls and previously analyzed patient specimens to control automated hematology analyzers. A minimum of 1 assayed control material (target value and limits defined) must be analyzed at least once every 24 hours to verify calibration. Thereafter, at least 2 specimens must be analyzed each shift to satisfy the quality control requirements. These 2 specimens may consist of 2 previously analyzed patient specimens, or 1 previously analyzed patient specimen and an assayed control, or 2 assayed controls. The HSQB interpretive guidelines make no mention of patient data algorithms, such as moving averages. For PT and aPTT, 2 levels of reference control are required per 8 hours of operation, and with each new vial of thromboplastin.[31]

REFERENCES

1. Bachner P: Quality assurance in hematology. In Howanitz PJ, Howanitz JH, eds: Laboratory quality assurance. McGraw-Hill, New York, 1987.

2. Cembrowski GS, Westgard JO: Quality control of multichannel analyzers: evaluation of Bull's algorithm. Am J Clin Pathol 83:337-345, 1985.

3. Britten GM, Brecher G, Johnson CA, Elashoff RM: Stability of blood on commonly used anticoagulants. Am J Clin Pathol 52:690-694, 1969.

4. Cembrowski GS, Lunetzky ES, Patrick CC, Wilson MK: Optimized quality control procedure for hematology analyzers using retained patient specimens. Am J Clin Pathol 89:203-210, 1988.

5. Carstairs KC, Peters E, Kuzin EJ: Development and description of the "random duplicates" method of quality control for a hematology laboratory. Am J Clin Pathol 67:379-385, 1977.

6. Riddick JH, Johnston CL: Hematology control using computerized range charts. Lab Med 3:32-34, 1972.

7. Orser B: Hematology quality control and the Coulter S+II. Am J Med Tech 49:643-647, 1983.

8. Weisbrot IM: Statistics for the clinical laboratory. JP Lippincott, Philadelphia, 1985, p 85.

9. Dorsey DB: Quality control in hematology. Am J Clin Pathol 40:457-464, 1963.

10. Bull BS, Elashoff RM, Heilbron DC, et al: A study of various estimators for the derivation of quality control procedures from patient erythrocyte indices. Am J Clin Pathol 61:473-481, 1974.

11. Bull BS, Korpman RA: Intra-laboratory quality control using patients' data. In Cavill I, ed, Methods in hematology, vol 4, Quality control. Churchill Livingstone, New York, 1982, pp 121-150.

12. Levy WC, Hay KL, Bull BS: Preserved blood versus patient data for quality control—Bull's algorithm revisited. Am J Clin Pathol 85:719-721, 1986.

13. Koepke JA, Protextor TJ: Quality assurance for multichannel hematology instruments, four years experience with patient mean erythrocyte indices. Am J Clin Pathol 75:28-33, 1981.

14. Cembrowski GS, Westgard JO: Quality control of multichannel hematology analyzers: evaluation of Bull's algorithm. Am J Clin Pathol 83: 337-345, 1985.

15. Lunetzky ES, Cembrowski GS: Performance characteristics of Bull's multirule algorithm for the quality control of multichannel hematology analyzers. Am J Clin Pathol 88:634-638, 1987.

16. Cembrowski GS, Schiller H, Wilson MK. Unpublished data.

17. Koepke JA, Dotson MA, Shifman MA: A critical evaluation of the manual/visual differential leukocyte counting method. Blood Cells 11:173-186, 1985.

18. Barnett CW: The unavoidable error in the differential count of the leukocytes of the blood. J Clin Invest 12:77-85, 1933.

19. Rumke CL: The statistically expected variability in differential leukocyte counting. Chapter IV. In Koepke JA, ed: The differential leukocyte count. College of American Pathologists, Skokie, Illinois, 1979.

20. Bull BS, Korpman RA: Characterization of the WBC differential count. Blood Cells 6:411-419, 1980.

21. Korpman RA, Bull BS: Whither the WBC differential?—Some alternatives. Blood Cells 6:421-429, 1980.

22. Pierre RV: Differential counting. In Koepke JA, ed: Laboratory hematology. Churchill Livingstone, New York, 1984, pp 973-997.

23. Dutcher TF: Leukocyte differentials. Are they worth the effort? Clin Lab Med 4(1):71-87, 1984.

24. Bull BS: Quality assurance strategies. In Koepke JA, ed: Laboratory hematology. Churchill Livingstone, New York, 1984, pp 999-1021.

25. Hackney JR, Hoste SL, Cembrowski, GS, Lunetzky ES. Quality control

of the automated screening differential. Presented at the Fall Meeting of the American Society of Clinical Pathologists, New Orleans, October 1987.

26. Cembrowski GS, Patrick CC: Use of a multi-rule control chart for the quality control of PT and aPTT. Presented at the Fall Meeting of the ASCP, Las Vegas, November 1985.

27. Hagemann P, Lunetzky ES, Cembrowski GS: Evaluation of the use of patient duplicates for the quality control of prothrombin time and activated partial thromboplastin time determinations: a computer simulation approach. Submitted for publication.

28. Joint Commission on Accreditation of Healthcare Organizations, Accreditation manual for hospitals. Chicago, 1989.

29. CAP Inspection Checklist, Hematology. College of American Pathologists Commission on Laboratory Accreditation, Skokie, Illinois, Spring 1987.

30. Health Care Financing Administration, United States Government, Interpretive guidelines for independent laboratories, Revision 189, p C-78.27. Washington, DC, June 1986.

31. Health Care Financing Administration, United States Government, Interpretive guidelines for independent laboratories, Revision 170, p C-79. Washington, DC, December 1984.

CHAPTER TEN

Computers in Quality Control

Computers have been used in the clinical laboratory since the 1960s.[1] One of the first implementations was at University of Wisconsin Hospitals, where analog signals from a Technicon Autoanalyzer (Technicon Instruments Corporation, Tarrytown, NY 10591) were transmitted to a computer via a retransmitting slidewire. The analyzer's sample carousel held a predefined sequence of standards, control samples, and patient samples. After analysis, the computer generated a working curve from the standard values and then calculated the control and patient results. Control values falling outside predefined control limits were flagged. Patient and control data were reviewed by the technologist, and if the control values were acceptable, patient test results were transcribed manually onto report forms for distribution to nursing stations. If the control values exceeded the control limits, the run was rejected. Patient results were not reported until the error was corrected and the samples were reanalyzed. This interaction between technologist and computer represented one of the first computer-aided quality control procedures in the clinical laboratory.

Further development of computerized quality control in the clinical laboratory lagged because of the limited capabilities of the earlier computers and the great emphasis placed on the acquisition, storage, and retrieval of patient data. The first computerized application of a multirule control procedure was not implemented in a laboratory information system (LIS) but in a stand-alone microcomputer using software dedicated to the analysis of quality control data entered manually.[2] Soon afterwards, analyzers began to perform their own quality control functions via self-contained software and hardware. In the last decade, instrument-based quality control systems have become more powerful and approach currently available microcomputer-based systems. The development of LIS-based quality control software has paralleled that of the instrument-based software; the newer systems are incorporating state of the art quality control practices. LIS-based systems may prove to be the major impetus for the general use of optimized quality control procedures.

With today's emphasis on laboratory economy and efficiency, even a small clinical laboratory generates enough data to justify computerized data collection, analysis, and reporting. Computerization can relieve the laboratorian of the tedious task of manually inspecting all incoming data. Instead, the computer continuously checks patient and control data; the laboratorian interprets the computer-generated error signals and uses the computer to record any corrective actions. The computer allows the laboratorian to rapidly react to error conditions even during peak workloads. The computer can standardize the manner in which data points are analyzed, recorded, summarized, and archived. Through the consistent treatment of the control data, a well-designed computerized quality control system will reinforce the quality control methods and policies practiced within a laboratory.

In this chapter we will describe examples of quality control software as it has been implemented in instrument-based, stand-alone microcomputer-based and LIS-based systems. Because computerized quality control is rapidly evolving, the descriptions of specific hardware, instruments, and software packages must be considered only as examples of what was available in 1988.

QUALITY CONTROL SYSTEM HARDWARE AND SOFTWARE

It is easy to devote excess attention to computer hardware considerations such as computer speed and disk capacity, and to lose sight of the qualitative aspects of a computerized system. Whenever evaluating a system, the following question should always be asked: "Does the software do its task well?" While computer hardware capabilities can place limitations on a quality control system, any hardware may be acceptable if it works reliably with the software, the system performs according to specification, and the specification is satisfactory to the user. Before acquiring any software or hardware, the prospective user should confirm that it already performs the intended functions in a laboratory of similar workload.

As computer technology advances, the power of computers and peripherals will increase and their costs will continue to decline. Already "desktop" computers have the power of earlier mainframe computers which cost 50 to 100 times more. Because of the rapidly changing computer technology, many different computers and computer systems will be available. The user should exercise caution whenever selecting hardware or software. Unique hardware and operating systems may not be easily replaced or upgraded, and if either the computer manufacturer or the software vendor suspends operation, the user may end up attempting to maintain an obsolete system.

INSTRUMENT-BASED SYSTEMS

With the availability of relatively inexpensive microprocessors, instrument manufacturers have been able to develop analyzers with expanded quality control functions. These functions are achieved through software operating on the same microprocessor used to regulate the instrument's operation or on a secondary microprocessor, which may consist of a personal computer attached to the main instrument. As a rule, the sophistication of instrument-based quality control functions are proportional to the complexity, speed, and size of the analyzer. Virtually all of today's instruments have an interface to allow connection to the LIS; their quality control functions may thus be supplemented or even replaced by the LIS. Examples of some instrument-based quality control systems are provided below.

Blood Gas Instrument Example

The IL-Fisher BGM, System 1312 Blood Gas Analyzer (Instrumentation Laboratory, Lexington, MA 02173) is a stand-alone laboratory instrument with moderate quality control capabilities. The system has a built-in data management system and can store up to 3000 patient records and 450 quality control results on a floppy disk. Control materials are identified by lot number and control results are subdivided into high, normal, and low control levels.

The quality control results for pH, PO_2, and PCO_2 can be printed or displayed. Control results can be organized by level of control and/or by work shift. The system can derive its own mean and standard deviation from the accumulated quality control data. While Levey-Jennings type control charts can be displayed or printed, the system does not test for control rule violations, but relies on visual inspection of the charts to detect out of control situations. This inspection can occur immediately after the control materials have been analyzed and allows prompt judgments about the state of control.

215

High-Speed Automated Chemistry Analyzer Example

The Paramax (American Dade Chemistry Systems, Irvine, CA 92718) represents a typical high-volume chemistry analyzer with sophisticated quality control functions. The Paramax has a control setup procedure in which the following information is specified: (1) the test name and the multirules to be applied to each test; (2) the names of the control materials and the analytes to be measured (tests) in each material; and (3) the expected mean and standard deviation of each test/control material combination. Specimens are identified by barcodes, and a unique barcode number is assigned to each different control material. Whenever a control material is to be sampled, a label with its barcode number is requested from Paramax and is used to identify the control specimen. After testing, results of any tests failing control rules are printed in red along with a failure report which lists the rules failed. The failure is automatically noted in the system Action Log file, where the operator can enter comments about the failure and corrective action taken. Levey-Jennings charts are available. The criteria for control result evaluation may be based on either the assigned mean and standard deviation or the entire lot-to-date mean and standard deviation calculated by Paramax.

Hematology Cell Counter Example

The Coulter S Plus IV (Coulter Electronics, Hialeah, FL 33012), a high-volume multichannel hematology analyzer, offers fairly standard quality control procedures for the setup and analysis of whole blood control data. It can process up to 9 different control materials. For each control material, the name of the control, lot number, expiration date, and local identification code are entered. Then for each control material and test, an assay range is entered. All of the results of any single control product can be presented either graphically or in a tabular format along with their target values. No multirule capability is offered. Additionally, a blood specimen can be analyzed several times with the average result used as 1 control value; this feature permits the use of retained patient specimens as secondary controls.

Bull's moving averages of the red cell indices are also computed and evaluated. The indices of the last 20 patient specimens are saved and averaged with Bull's algorithm to yield a correction factor which is added to the previous Bull's mean to yield a new mean. The latest mean of the indices is then saved along with the previous 19 means. The means for the various indices can be displayed in a tabular format

216

or else graphically to show trends. Bull's means are flagged if they fall outside their 3% limits. Individual patient values which are very low and incompatible with life are recognized as washes and automatically deleted from the values used to derive the patient means. When a patient specimen is deleted, the patient batch is resized downward rather than collecting more data for the Bull's algorithm calculation.

MICROCOMPUTER-BASED SYSTEMS

Microcomputer quality control systems are usually stand-alone and are not as complex as their LIS counterparts. As a result, most microcomputer quality control systems require minimal training and computer experience. Instructions for data entry, report generation, and file manipulation are provided in the instruction manual. Reference to this manual should be infrequent if the user interface has been well designed. However, most microcomputer quality control programs do require the assistance of someone with microcomputer experience, because confusion often arises during the system initialization and the first attempts at running the program.

Table 10-1, modified after Stewart and Oxford,[3] compares the features of 4 different microcomputer-based quality control systems. One of the systems, QAS Today, is described more completely in the next section. Most of the microcomputer-based programs offer, as part of the overall package, the ability for a laboratory to regularly compare the analytical performance of its instruments to identical instruments in other laboratories analyzing similar lots of control material. The monthly means and standard deviations of control results are sent to a central facility via modem or mail, and each user laboratory's within-instrument means and standard deviations are compared to aggregate means and standard deviations of specific instrument/control combinations. A summary of the comparisons, also known as a peer report, is returned to the user. The use of these peer reports is somewhat limited as they permit only retrospective review of the findings.

Microcomputers can perform nearly immediate quality control evaluations of instruments and methods which produce small numbers of control data. Even when used with these methods, the microcomputer can slow a laboratory's operation. Virtually all of the current general purpose microcomputer quality control programs only allow data entry via the keyboard. Because data cannot be transmitted directly from the analyzer to the microcomputer, delay is incurred during the data entry step. Most of these systems cannot support multiple users simultaneously, and delay is experienced if more than 1 user

Table 10-1 Summary of example microcomputer-based quality control software.

Program Name	ACLAIM-QAP	LabTrack QC-2	QAS Today	QMS
Supplier	Dade	Fisher	CAP	Prism Associates
control levels	3	6	6	4
Data entry:				
Single point entry	yes	yes	yes	yes
Batch entry	yes	yes	yes	yes
Panel definition	no	yes	yes	yes
Statistics available:				
L-J charts	yes	yes	yes	yes
Mean, SD (MTD)	yes	yes	yes	yes
Mean, SD (LTD)	yes	yes	yes	yes
Multirule	yes	yes	yes	yes
Cusum	no	yes	no	yes
Trigg's trend analysis	no	yes	no	yes
Mean check across	no	no	yes	yes
Lot change routine	yes	no	yes	yes
Password security	yes	yes	none	yes
Peer review	yes	no	yes	via CAP
Telecommunications (Modem use)	yes	no	yes	yes
Training/Help:				
User manual	yes	yes	yes	yes
Training sessions	yes	yes	no	pending
Help screens	yes	yes	no	yes
1-800 assistance	yes	yes	yes	no

Abbreviations: L-J = Levey-Jennings, MTD = month to date, LTD = lot to date
Modified with permission. From Stewart and Oxford. J Med Tech 2:621-628, 1985.

requires access to the system at the same time. Further delays occur when the calculations or quality control rules are complex. While multiple microcomputer systems will speed the quality control processing of busy laboratory sections and enable remotely located sections to computerize their quality control, they will impede the centralization of the quality control information.

High-volume instruments do not lend themselves to stand-alone microcomputer quality control. Keyboard entry of the 300 control results produced hourly by the SMAC (Technicon) will result in either delayed reporting of patient data or in retrospective quality control. Fortunately most high-volume instruments, including the SMAC II, can now perform their own quality control, and the microcomputer quality control program simply accepts summary statistics from the instrument-based quality control system and then forwards them to the appropriate peer review facility.

Because of the delays in data entry and analysis, some laboratories have adopted an "after the fact" use of these microcomputer systems. Control results are generated and inspected manually, usually without the advantage of multirule techniques. These same quality control results are subsequently entered into the microcomputer quality control system, and the automated quality control analysis is performed long after the patient results have been reported. Although the quality control system is not used to ascertain accuracy and precision before reporting of the patient results, centralization of quality control data and peer review are still achieved.

Microcomputer-Based System Example

The College of American Pathologists (CAP) developed the QAS Today program to support its Quality Assurance Service (QAS) program. Table 10–1 summarizes the features of QAS Today. While there is no fee for the use of the microcomputer program, there is a charge for maintaining peer-review files on the main CAP computer system and for report generation. Fees depend on the number of methods and control materials monitored. QAS will accept information from any user regardless of the method of analysis or brand of control material; however, the peer review is of little use if unpopular methods or control materials are used.

QAS Today can be used with multiple computer operating systems. The software is menu driven with menus dividing the program into the following functional units: initialization, data entry, data analysis, and data transmission. When the program is initialized, the user sets up an individual file for each control material/method combination. QAS Today can accept up to 6 levels of control material per method for across material statistical analysis. The following parameters must be specified for each file: file number (for future access to the data), analyte name, measurement unit, number of decimal places, assay value of the control material (entered if assayed material is used), code for the control material, text description of the control material, level of control material (refers to high, normal, or low concentration), and file type. The file type can be either a single point or multipoint file. In a *single point* file, single control values are entered and immediately evaluated. In a *multipoint file*, 2 or more control values are entered for a level of control material at 1 time.

QAS Today allows flexibility in the setting of control limits. The mean and standard deviation, from which the control limits are usually derived, can be calculated from all of the available control data for the most recent lot number, or from any specified time interval, including the last month's. "Fixed" limits, usually based on medical need, can be used instead of statistical limits. The final step in set up is specifying the control rules and the different levels of control materials which would be evaluated by the rules.

After initialization, the files are ready for data entry. As the data are entered, the program checks for absurd values and the correct number of decimal places. The user must initiate statistical review after data entry. The program analyzes the data, prints out whether the review was successful or not, and if an error condition exists. The system can display or print control charts. QAS Today, like most of the other microcomputer quality control programs, can print these control charts with or without data points.

Files can be set up to accept statistical summaries of the data. This is useful when such information is already provided, either by the laboratory computer or instrument. One summary file is created for each control material/method combination, and the following data are entered: number of controls analyzed, mean, and standard deviation.

LABORATORY INFORMATION SYSTEM–BASED SYSTEMS

LIS-based quality control systems have major advantages over stand-alone, microcomputer-based systems. The quality control procedures implemented on the LIS can be standardized throughout the laboratory. The best LIS-based quality control systems have been designed to be integrated into the laboratory's work flow and have increased laboratory efficiency. Quality control data entry and review for run acceptance occur during the same terminal session that patient data are entered. Any LIS terminal can function as a quality control workstation at any time, thus guaranteeing ready availability of quality control functions. Quality control data may be directly transmitted from automated instruments online to the LIS. Even if an automated instrument performs its own quality control, the LIS can centralize the quality control information. For each instrument, the laboratory has the option of using that instrument's internal quality control programs or that of the LIS, or a combination of the two. One of the authors' hematology laboratories uses the hematology analyzers's Bull's algorithm for evaluating patient data and the LIS-based Westgard multirules for evaluating the whole blood control data.

LIS quality control analysis can provide immediate feedback and control. If patient and control values are transmitted promptly to the LIS, quality control processing occurs immediately and runs are rejected before patient results are released to reporting stations. Documentation can be dramatically improved and centralized via a LIS. One of the authors' laboratories has achieved a "paperless" quality control system by combining coded and free text comment modifiers with the quality control results in its Flexilab (Sunquest Information Systems, Tucson, AZ 85710) LIS. Corrective action for control rule failures, reagent lot changes, and effective dates of procedure changes are documented in this manner.

Compared to the microcomputer quality control vendor, the LIS vendor has usually demonstrated a greater commitment to guarantee acceptable system performance. Most LIS vendors provide training, technical assistance, and some software customization. Decisions about quality control procedures are usually made during the preinstallation phase by the laboratory with assistance from the vendor's installation specialists.

A LIS has disadvantages, the main one being cost. Expenditures for hardware and software are very high, with typical systems for moderate-sized hospitals costing between $500,000 and $1,000,000. LIS development and installation costs are significant and cannot be spread over large volumes of sales, as can other types of computer systems. Some LIS quality control programs are clumsy, tedious, and ineffective. State of the art quality control procedures were developed after many of the current LISs were designed; thus, some quality control software is an afterthought which is not fully integrated into some systems.

Quality control software constitutes an essential component of the modern LIS. We believe that a laboratory's quality control functions and quality control database should reside in the LIS. In this way, operators need to learn the idiosyncrasies of only the LIS quality control software, instead of the individual peculiarities of quality control software on multiple instruments, microcomputers, and the LIS. When quality control functions are performed by the LIS, only 1 database is needed for the storage of control results and ranges. Furthermore, the LIS can most effectively perform quality control procedures relying on patient data, eg, delta checks.

Many laboratories operate without a LIS, while others have a LIS which does not offer extensive quality control features. Some LISs are near the end of their useful lives, and it is not economically feasible for vendors to design comprehensive quality control functions for them. The system software that is used by some current LISs makes the addition of new quality control features prohibitively expensive in terms of programmer and computer time. Thus, many laboratories will continue to rely on microcomputer and instrument-based quality control software to automate most of their quality control procedures.

There are several popular commercially available LISs with extensive quality control capabilities. They are well designed for functionality and efficiency. Some other systems have even more capability, but these are unique systems developed by individuals with special interest in quality control. These systems are not readily transferable to other sites.

No comparison of commercial LIS quality control software features is provided in this book; LIS quality control programs are evolving, making any published comparison outdated in just a few months. One feature, peer review, will be briefly discussed. Peer review is not usually part of the LIS's quality control functions. If a laboratory with a LIS participates in peer review, end-of-month mean, standard deviation, and number of control results are usually submitted by mail for each method/test/control combination. A few LISs already have the capability to download files and reports to microcomputers.

LIS-Based System Example

Labcom+ (Laboratory Consulting Incorporated, Madison, WI 53701) was developed by the vendor and the staff of the University of Wisconsin Hospitals Clinical Laboratories. Quality control results are stored in files based on the analyte, test method, and control product employed. When quality control record files are initialized, single control rules or multirule type control rules are selected by the user. Any combination of the standard rules can be selected. Quality control rules can be applied within and across runs, within control material and across material. Range rules are not permitted across runs, thus reducing the incidence of false rejection. Any rule can be selected as either a warning or rejection signal. During data entry, Labcom+ checks for the entry of absurd values, panic values, and appropriate number of decimal places. A program module is available to perform delta checks on patient values.

Up to 4 separate sets of control rules can be chosen, corresponding to different modes of quality control analysis: (1) method startup, (2) routine operation, (3) emergency use, and (4) retrospective analysis.

Method startup mode is used either at startup or after maintenance. Analytical error is more prevalent in these situations, and it is important to detect and correct errors before a method is used routinely. (See Chapter 8 for discussion of multistage quality control.) Quality control rules are chosen with high sensitivity (eg, 1_{2s} for rejection). Methods that pass these rules may then be used for patient specimen analysis. In the *routine mode* rules are chosen so that false rejection is decreased. There is an *emergency mode* which is used when an infrequently used method must be employed, eg, when a primary analyzer malfunctions. A high probability of error detection is required to assure the quality of the alternate method. While the method startup mode can be used, the emergency mode offers more flexibility. In the *retrospective mode*, usually performed at the end of day, the entire day's quality control results are reanalyzed, with calibration checks made, and additional rules are used which are sensitive to longer term variation (eg, 4_{1s} and 10_x). The additional rules are employed retrospectively as warning rules, rather than rejection rules, and can be used to detect problems which can be corrected so that they are not carried over to the next day.

IMPLEMENTING COMPUTERIZED QUALITY CONTROL

Regardless of whether the laboratory automates quality control via instrument, microprocessor, or LIS, implementation of an automated quality control system requires the education of all individuals who use the software. This effort will far exceed that of introducing a new analytical method, where only a few people must be trained. Everyone must understand the new quality control process. At least 2 individuals are required per laboratory section who are knowledgeable about the operation of the quality control software. These 2 key personnel must understand the dictionary definition procedure for setting up quality control rules and limits for each method/test/control. For poorly designed systems, these individuals might need to be familiar with system-specific features, including operating system, instruction sets, and file manipulation. The quality control personnel must assemble many data to initialize the quality control system: analyte, control name, control lot number, assigned mean, assigned standard deviation, control rules. They must be able to instruct the other workers how to enter and edit data, produce quality control reports and charts, initiate data analysis, and prepare data summaries for peer review. These personnel must have an aptitude for these tasks and an active interest, otherwise problems can arise. In 1 study, technologists' lack of familiarity with microcomputers was the most frequent problem encountered in the implementation of a microcomputer quality control program.[4]

LIMITATIONS

Computerized quality control has certain disadvantages. Some personnel demonstrate anxiety when working with computers. This "computer fear" must be allayed as it can hinder the transition to successful computerized quality control. Review of quality control data resident in the computer may not be as convenient as review of control charts which are manually prepared. Computerization will not completely obviate the requirement for manual quality control procedures as they must be available during computer failure. Computerization requires the periodic duplication and storage of quality control data to prevent their loss during computer failure.

Computerization can result in virtually unalterable quality control systems. This inflexibility arises from deficiencies in program design and implementation. Some laboratorians regard the use of a computerized quality control system as a passive process in which their input is minimal. Such attitudes, if pervasive, will result in poor understanding of the quality control process and flawed quality control practices. To prevent these attitudinal problems, the limitations that the computer software impose on the quality control procedures must be recognized. The use of an automated quality control system is no substitute for a thorough understanding of the principles and practices of quality control.

FUTURE DEVELOPMENTS

As the cost of computer hardware continues to decrease, it is likely that cost of the hardware component of the LIS will also drop and its capabilities will increase. A central LIS coprocessor with a direct instrument interface will become a commonly accepted approach for acquiring patient and quality control data. Such an arrangement would preserve the centralization of the quality control functions and database. From a management perspective, the centralization and resulting uniformity of all quality control functions are the most significant features of LIS-based quality control.

For those laboratories which are unable to obtain LIS-based quality control systems, instrument- and stand-alone microprocessor-based systems are preferable to no system at all. The performance of these latter 2 systems continues to improve due to the increasing power and decreasing price of microprocessor-driven computer systems. The quality control capabilities of the instrument- and microcomputer-based systems will approach those offered by the best of the LIS-based systems.

With such arrangements, quality control can be done by either the instrument or the LIS. Both approaches, the centralized large computer and the instrument- and microcomputer-based system, have advantages. In the latter system, the immediate quality control functions, eg, those seen in the startup and routine mode, might be done more readily on the instrument, and retrospective quality control on the LIS. Quality control functions using patient data would better be accomplished by the LIS.

Software exists to accomplish most of the quality control procedures described in this book; however, only subsets of these procedures are available in any single system. A recent survey of users of the MEDLAB LIS (3M Health Information Systems, Salt Lake City, Utah 84107) indicated a strong desire to have all of the modern quality control procedures available.[5] Development is required of all vendors to increase the repertoire of quality control procedures.

The other principal requirement of laboratory quality control software is an improved computer-user interface. Clumsy features can be demonstrated in all current laboratory quality control software. In other fields, state of the art software has been produced with the user interface designed for maximum productivity and minimum effort.[6] Electronic pointers, pull-down menus, "windowing," and icon-driven software allow individuals to use computer systems efficiently and bypass the large amount of detail formerly required. High priority should be placed on implementing these features in quality control software.

REFERENCES

1. Hicks GP, Evenson MA, Gieschen MM, Larson FC: On-line data acquisition in the clinical laboratory. In Stacy RW, Waxman BD, eds: Computers in Biomedical Research. Academic Press, New York, 1969, pp 15-53.

2. Westgard JO: Better quality control through micro-computers. Diag Med 5:60-74, 1982.

3. Stewart CE, Oxford BS: Quality assurance programs and quality control data management. J Med Tech 2:621-628, 1985.

4. Kafka M, Howanitz P, DiSilvio T, Veil J, Kryzak P: Development and

implementation of QAS Today, a quality control software program. Clin Chem 30(6):959, 1984.

5. Martin PL, Robb D: Quality control questionnaire distributed to the Medlab Users' Group, Fall 1986. Findings presented at the Medlab Users' Group Meeting, Salt Lake City, January 1987.

6. Simpson: Programming the IBM PC user interface. McGraw-Hill, New York, 1986.

CHAPTER ELEVEN

External Proficiency Testing (Interlaboratory Quality Control)

ORIGINS OF INTERLABORATORY SURVEYS

Whenever a new analytical method is evaluated, both its precision and accuracy must be determined. Precision is estimated from replicate analyses; accuracy is assessed by testing patient specimens with the new method and a reference (comparative) method. The reference method can be performed in the same laboratory or in another laboratory. Once the new method is used routinely, comparisons to the reference method are usually discontinued. The laboratory must then rely on its reference sample quality control procedures to detect deterioration of a method's performance. Without comparison to alternate or reference methods, inaccuracies in the analytical method may develop, due to slow drifts or calibration problems.

Laboratories can participate in interlaboratory surveys, and periodically compare their methods to other laboratories. In these surveys, identical specimens are sent to all participants for analysis, and each laboratory's results are assessed according to their agreement with the group mean or to results obtained by analysis with a reference method. This type of quality control, referred to as *external quality control, external proficiency testing, proficiency testing* or *interlaboratory quality control*, originated in 1946 with Belk and Sunderman, who submitted samples from the same serum pool to 59 Pennsylvania hospital laboratories to check the analytical accuracy for common chemical analytes.[1] Their initial results demonstrated large differences between laboratories, and a need to reduce these differences. One year later, the College of American Pathologists (CAP) began voluntary interlaboratory chemistry surveys.[2] During the late 40s and early 50s additional voluntary interlaboratory testing programs were developed by CAP, other professional societies, and state and municipal health departments.[3,4] These programs emphasized self analysis and self improvement by the participants. Laboratory directors who participated in these programs were expected to evaluate the proficiency test results and, if necessary, initiate corrective action. The objectives of these early interlaboratory surveys were to profile laboratory testing on the national level, stimulate interest in better techniques and methods, and to diminish interlaboratory variability through education.[5]

REGULATORY/ACCREDITATION APPLICATION

The voluntary nature of the interlaboratory survey programs changed with the enactment of Medicare in 1966,[6] and the Clinical Laboratory Improvement Act (CLIA) of 1967.[7] Through these laws, the federal government mandated "successful" participation in interlaboratory surveys. The federal regulatory agencies rationalized that the same information used by laboratory directors to evaluate the quality of their laboratory results could be used for regulatory (certification of quality) purposes. As a result, laboratories not performing adequately in proficiency testing were denied licensure under CLIA or by Medicare. The primary motive for participating in proficiency testing was shifted from quality and self improvement to regulation.

Subsequent medicare amendments extended health insurance to the aged and established inspection and quality control requirements for independent laboratories. Laboratories involved in interstate commerce were mandated by CLIA to participate in a proficiency testing program. Compliance with Medicare's proficiency testing requirement could be met through participation in approved federal, state, or professional programs. For example, hospitals which participated in federally approved proficiency testing programs (such as CAP's) were exempted from participation in federal government sponsored proficiency testing programs.[7,8] While requirements for both Medicare and CLIA have undergone multiple reinterpretations and revisions since 1968, every clinical laboratory in the United States of America is now required to participate in at least one interlaboratory proficiency testing program as a condition of licensure under state, CLIA, Medicare, or professional requirements such as those of CAP or the Joint Commission for the Accreditation of Health Care Organizations (JCAHO). Interlaboratory proficiency testing has become a routine component in the clinical laboratory's quality assurance program.[9]

The educational intent of proficiency testing programs has been compromised as the regulatory component has grown. The fundamental premise of proficiency testing as a regulatory-licensure requirement is that if a laboratory performs acceptably in a proficiency testing program, it also analyzes patient samples correctly. However, the question remains: "Does performance in interlaboratory programs represent routine intralaboratory performance?" It is reasonable to assume that proficiency testing samples receive preferential treatment when accreditation or licensure is at issue. Most regulators and professional organizations recognize that the performance measured by proficiency testing is indicative of the "best" that the laboratory can do and not of its routine performance.[10]

PROFICIENCY TESTING PROGRAMS

Proficiency testing programs, both regulatory and voluntary, are available from a variety of sources. Many of these programs are designed to be both educational and acceptable for regulatory purposes. The largest interlaboratory proficiency testing programs, those of CAP, serve both functions, as do the programs of the American Association of Bioanalysts (AAB). Most accrediting organizations and state regulations require laboratories to participate in proficiency testing programs for tests that they perform. Most states accept CAP and/or the AAB programs for meeting licensure requirements. Proficiency testing programs are offered by the Centers for Disease Control. Some states, most notably New York, Wisconsin, and Pennsylvania, offer regulatory proficiency testing programs as requirements for laboratory licensure. The American Association for Clinical Chemistry (Drug Analyses), the American Thoracic Society (Blood Gases), American Association of Blood Banks (Donor Testing), and other professional organizations provide specialized programs.

More recently, manufacturers of some instrument systems and quality control products have begun to provide interlaboratory quality assurance programs. These "manufacturer" programs are currently not accepted by the regulatory agencies for licensure purposes, but provide valuable interinstrumental comparisons, as well as assessment of intralaboratory precision. They are currently the only true voluntary interlaboratory quality assurance programs. If more laboratories adopt manufacturer offered programs, they may eventually be accepted for regulatory purposes.

Most proficiency testing programs provide results to regulatory agencies, in accordance with the requests of the participants. The regulatory agency may follow up immediately on "unacceptable" results, and may provide further followup with an on site inspection and examination of the intralaboratory quality control. During on site inspection, the inspection team reviews and evaluates the laboratory's proficiency testing performance and corrective actions taken in response to proficiency testing results.

Logistics

All proficiency testing programs follow a fairly uniform sequence:

1. Uniform samples are distributed to participants on a scheduled basis.
2. Participants reconstitute samples, perform testing, record results, identify methods, and return results to central facility.
3. Data are coded and processed at central facility.
4. Results are graded based on program-selected criteria (or criteria required by federal regulation); results are usually grouped by methodology where possible, thus yielding a relatively homogeneous subpopulation for comparison.
5. Results and grades are distributed to participants and to regulatory agencies, if required.
6. Results are evaluated by the participating laboratories for quality assurance purposes.

Proficiency specimens are usually distributed quarterly with 1 to 5 samples in each shipment, although the frequency of distribution can be as often as monthly. Protracted turnaround times present a major problem to program organizers; turnaround times can be drawn out by many factors, including sample distribution, the run frequencies in the participating laboratories, result reporting, result processing, and grade distribution. Unfortunately, as turnaround times lengthen, the data's usefulness to the participants is diminished.

Samples

The ideal proficiency testing sample should imitate a recently collected specimen. Because of the need for large, stable, homogeneous pools of material and for wide ranges of analyte concentrations, proficiency testing specimens are often composed of a nonhuman matrix and contain exogenous additives. Many clinical chemistry proficiency testing specimens are lyophilized, and thus require special handling, including reconstitution with specific volumes of diluent. These factors increase interlaboratory variation. Samples may thus lack uniformity because of variation during the processes of manufacturing, filling, mailing, storage, reconstitution, and other preanalytical handling. The statistical impact of this interlaboratory variation is analogous to the impact of between-run variation on reference sample quality control procedures (see Chapter 6).

Samples often contain nonhuman components, many of which react differently when used with analytical methodologies which have been developed specifically for human specimens. As a result, interlaboratory variation always includes error which is due to the sample itself. Moreover, atypical sample matrices can cause great differences in interinstrumental or intermethod performance. Unless these matrix effects are fully understood, it is difficult to establish relationships between different analytical systems.

PERFORMANCE LIMITS AND GRADING

Since 1966, CAP has used the range specified by the mean ± 2S limits, where the mean is the interlaboratory mean and S is the interlaboratory standard deviation, to define acceptable proficiency testing performance. During the data reduction process, the mean and standard deviation are determined. Any observations which exceed mean ± 3S limits are omitted, and the mean and standard deviation are recalculated to derive a "trimmed" mean and S.[11,12] From 1966 to 1969, CAP survey results within mean ± 2S were classified as "acceptable"; those exceeding ± 2S were "not acceptable."[11] From 1970 to the present, "good" results have been within ± 1S, "acceptable" within ± 2S, and "unacceptable" beyond ± 2S.[13,14] The Clinical Laboratories Improvement Act has defined acceptable proficiency testing performance as being within ± 2S.[7] The Health Care Financing Administration defines unsuccessful performance in a proficiency testing program as 3 unsatisfactory results or 3 unsatisfactory results in 4 shipments.[15]

Most programs assign grades to laboratory results to enable rapid evaluation of performance. CAP uses a calculated grading parameter called the standard deviation index or interval (SDI):[13]

$$\text{SDI} = (\text{laboratory value} - \text{group mean})/\text{group } S.$$

The interlaboratory group mean and S are calculated from a homogeneous group of instruments or methods. The SDI value is the number of group standard deviations by which an individual laboratory's result differs from the group mean. SDIs within ± 2 SDI indicate that the result falls within the group mean ± 2 group S limits. Values outside the group mean ± 2 SDI limits are not acceptable and indicate a need for investigation, and possibly a failure (if done for regulatory purposes). Investigative actions can include review of intralaboratory quality control, retesting of the proficiency testing sample, or analysis of a followup proficiency testing sample.

When ± 2 SDI limits are used, 5% of the results are defined as unacceptable according to statistical theory, in the absence of any error except the inherent random error of the laboratories. When statistical limits such as ± 2S are applied to precise and accurate instruments, the small interlaboratory Ss will result in a narrow range of acceptable performance. Consequently, laboratories with numerically small errors will often fail proficiency testing. Laboratories with less precise or accurate systems, and thus with large interlaboratory standard deviations, often pass proficiency testing with numerically large errors. As a result, many proficiency testing programs are abandoning statistical limits and are adopting the use of fixed limits.

The fixed limit approach can counteract the effects of overly stringent or lenient performance requirements created by interlaboratory group Ss.[16] Fixed limits are conceptually simple; they correspond to a fixed specific interval expressed as a percentage of the participant's group mean or target value. Gilbert and Platt[17] first applied fixed limits to calcium and potassium results in the 1978 CAP Interlaboratory Survey Program. More recently, CAP has adopted fixed limits to evaluate the performance of participants for commonly tested chemistry, hematology, and blood gas analytes.[14,18] These fixed limits are shown in Table 11–1, and are compared to medical usefulness limits. Fixed limits are not affected by state of the art performance, and are not dependent on the PT group performance. They make no assumptions about the source of error, ie, systematic (bias) or random error (imprecision). Fixed limits can easily be compared to total intralaboratory analytical error. A laboratory result within the fixed limit passes proficiency testing; a result exceeding it fails. Whenever the fixed limit is less than twice the group standard deviation, more results are classified as unacceptable than when the ± 2 SDI criterion is used.

At a minimum, proficiency testing criteria should warn the laboratory and the regulatory agencies when intralaboratory performance is not meeting patient needs. Proficiency testing, however, should also not fail good laboratories.

RESPONSE OF PERFORMANCE LIMIT GRADING TO INTRALABORATORY PERFORMANCE CHARACTERISTICS

The criterion selected for evaluation of intralaboratory performance strongly influences a proficiency testing program's ability to distinguish

Table 11-1   Fixed limits for evaluation of CAP survey results.

Constituent	E_a, $2CV_a$	Survey Allowable Error
Blood Gas[a,b]		
pH	0.008 at 7.35	0.03
	0.012 at 7.45	
pO$_2$	10 mm Hg at 80 mm Hg	7.5% or 5 mm Hg
pCO$_2$	6 mm Hg at 35, 50 mm Hg	7.5% or 3 mm Hg
Chemistry[a,b]		
albumin	0.5 g/dL at 3.5 g/dL	0.2 g/dL or 6.7%
calcium	0.5 mg/dL at 11.0 mg/dL	1.0 mg/dL
chloride	4 mmol/L at 90, 110 mmol/L	5.0 mmol/L
cholesterol	40 mg/dL at 250 mg/dL	15%
creatinine	0.3 mg/dL at 2.0 mg/dL	6.7% or 0.2 mg/dL
glucose	10 mg/dL at 100 mg/dL	6.0 mg/dL or 13.3%
phosphorus	0.5 mg/dL at 4.5 mg/dL	0.3 mg/dL or 10.7%
potassium	0.5 mmol/L at 3,6 mmol/L	0.5 mmol/L
sodium	4 mmol/L at 130, 150 mmol/L	4.0 mmol/L
total protein	0.6g/dL at 7.0 g/dL	5.8%
urea	4 mg/dL at 27 mg/dL	8.8% or 2 mg N/dL
uric acid	1 mg/dL at 6.0 mg/dL	16.7%
Hematology[c,d]		
hematocrit	10.8%	3 SDI or 6%
hemoglobin	7.2%	3 SDI or 5%
platelet count		3 SDI or 25%
RBC		3 SDI or 6%
WBC	32.8%	3 SDI or 10%

Abbreviations: E_a = allowable error.

[a] Allowable error from Barnett,[28] derived by multiplying allowable standard deviation times 2 (see Chapter 5).

[b] CAP limit for acceptable performance for blood gas and chemistry analytes is whichever is greater when both concentration and percentage are given.

[c] Allowable error from Skendzel, Barnett and Platt,[29] derived as above.

[d] CAP limit for acceptable performance for hematology is lesser of the percentage or SDI terms.

Reproduced with permission. From Interlaboratory comparison program: CAP surveys manual, section III, chemistry. College of American Pathologists, Skokie, IL, 1987, pp 9–10. And from Interlaboratory comparison program: CAP surveys manual, section II hematology-coagulation/clinical microscopy. College of American Pathologists, Skokie, IL, 1987, p 15.

good and deficient intralaboratory performance. Ehrmeyer and Laessig have used computer simulation techniques[19,20] to quantify the effect of intralaboratory performance characteristics, imprecision (coefficient of variation or CV) and inaccuracy (bias), on the ability of proficiency testing to characterize intralaboratory performance correctly.[21,22] They studied both statistical limit and fixed limit criteria. The computer simulation program is similar to that described in Chapter 3. It uses a gaussian random number generator which simulates the effect of intralaboratory variation in a population of many laboratories, each with its own intralaboratory bias and CV.[23] The program simulates multiple PT surveys and determines the frequency with which results from a laboratory with a particular CV-bias combination exceed the limit selected as the criterion for acceptable performance.

± 2 SDI Limits

Ehrmeyer and Laessig used the proficiency testing simulation program to evaluate the effectiveness of ± 2 SDI limits. Table 11–2 shows representative output from their evaluation, the percentage of laboratory results from laboratories with specified CV-bias combinations which fail a proficiency testing program when the interlaboratory standard deviation is 5% and the group mean is 100. Table 11–2 is divided into acceptable and unacceptable laboratories with acceptable performance being defined as having 5% or less of proficiency test results exceeding ± 2S limits. Thus a laboratory with a CV of 4% and no internal bias will have 2% of its proficiency testing results outside the ± 2S limits. A laboratory with a CV of 7% and an internal bias of 6% will have 31% of its proficiency testing results exceeding the ± 2S limits.

Fixed Limits

Ehrmeyer and Laessig also evaluated the effectiveness of fixed limits as grading criteria. They used probability calculations to simulate various combinations of intralaboratory bias and imprecision. Table 11–3 shows the percentage of proficiency testing results failing a ± 10% fixed limit for various intralaboratory bias and CV values.[24] Ideally, selection of the fixed limit and the acceptable outlier rate should be based on medical usefulness criteria (see Chapter 5). In Table 11–3, an acceptable outlier rate of 5% has been selected, and Table 11–3 has been divided into laboratories which have 5% or less unacceptable results and those which have more than 5%.

Table 11–2 Percentage of occasions on which PT results exceed survey mean ± 2S limits for various combinations of intralaboratory CV and bias relative to grand mean.

Intralaboratory CV, %		0	1	2	3	4	5	6	7	8	9	10
10		30	30	30	31	36	38	41	42	46	50	52
9		25	25	26	26	31	35	38	42	43	48	51
8		20	20	22	24	26	32	34	38	41	46	50
7		14	16	17	20	22	24	31	35	38	45	49
6		10	11	12	14	16	20	26	32	37	44	49
5		5	6	6	9	12	15	21	28	35	41	48
4		2	2	2	5	7	11	15	21	30	38	48
3		0	0	1	2	3	6	9	15	25	34	47
2		0	0	0	0	0	1	3	7	15	28	45
1		0	0	0	0	0	0	0	0	4	14	39

Intralaboratory Bias, %

Note: Assumes PT population group mean of 100 and group CV = 5%.

A laboratory having any of the CV-bias combinations shown in the lower left sector of Tables 11–2 and 11–3 will produce results which exceed either ± 2S limits or ± 10% error limits, respectively, 5% or less of the time. Since the lower left sector comprises laboratories with intralaboratory CV-bias combinations compatible with good performance, it would be preferable that these laboratories never fail proficiency testing.

Because laboratories with any of the CV-bias combinations outside of the lower left sector of Tables 11–2 and 11–3 would report results with excessive error more than 5% of the time, their intralaboratory performance can then be defined as bad performance, not producing medically useful data. It would be desirable that laboratories with any of these CV-bias combinations should fail the proficiency testing program 100% of the time.

EFFICIENCY OF PROFICIENCY TESTING PROGRAMS

The capabilities of a proficiency testing program can be evaluated in terms of predictive values and efficiencies. Laboratories whose CV-bias combinations fall in the lower left sectors of Tables 11–2 and 11–

235

Table 11–3 Percentage of occasions on which PT results exceed grand mean ± 10% limits for various combinations of intralaboratory CV and bias relative to grand mean.

Intralaboratory CV, %	0	1	2	3	4	5	6	7	8	9	10
10	32	32	33	34	36	38	40	43	46	49	52
9	27	27	28	29	31	34	37	40	43	47	51
8	21	21	23	24	27	30	33	37	41	46	51
7	15	16	17	19	22	25	29	34	39	45	50
6	10	10	11	14	17	21	26	31	37	43	50
5	5	5	6	9	12	16	21	27	34	42	50
4	1	2	2	4	7	11	16	23	31	40	50
3	0	0	0	1	2	5	9	16	25	37	50
2	0	0	0	0	0	1	2	7	16	31	50
1	0	0	0	0	0	0	0	0	2	16	50

Intralaboratory Bias, %

Note: Assumes PT population group mean of 100.

3, and who are graded as passing, may be classified true negatives (TN), while the laboratories in this sector who do not pass proficiency testing are false positives (FP). Carrying the analogy one step further, those laboratories in the other sector with CV-bias combinations not meeting the criteria for acceptable performance and correctly characterized as failing are the true positives (TP), whereas those declared to "pass" are the false negatives (FN). The overall performance of any proficiency testing scheme is characterized by its efficiency:

$$\text{Efficiency} = \frac{TP + TN}{TP + TN + FP + FN}.$$

Efficiency is affected by the prevalence of poorly performing laboratories in the population. Table 11–4 shows the effectiveness of different fixed limits (2% to 20%) as evaluation criteria for a proficiency testing program when good performance is defined as having results exceeding ± 10% limits less than 5% of the time, and the prevalence of poorly performing laboratories is 10%. A fixed limit of ± 2% fails 70% of the good laboratories and 86% of the bad laboratories, for an overall efficiency of 36%. As the fixed limit expands, more of the good laboratories are passed, but fewer of the bad laboratories fail. At a fixed

Table 11–4 Ability of PT programs using fixed limits to characterize intralaboratory performance correctly (good performance defined as ≤ 5% of results which exceed mean ± 10% limits; assume 10% prevalence of bad labs).

	% Correctly Identified		Efficiency
Fixed Limits	Good Labs	Bad Labs	(10% prevalence)
2%	30%	86%	36%
3%	48%	79%	51%
4%	62%	72%	63%
5%	75%	65%	74%
10%	100%	31%	93%
15%	100%	8%	91%
20%	100%	2%	90%

limit of 10%, 100% of the good laboratories pass, and 31% of the bad laboratories fail, and efficiency is 93%.

Whether proficiency testing programs use ± 2S limits or fixed limits, maximum efficiencies achievable are essentially equal to the prevalence of good laboratories. Both types of limits, when small, mislabel many good laboratories as bad, and when large, fail to detect bad laboratories. The situation is directly analogous to the inability of quality control rules to detect small increases in error when few control samples are tested, as demonstrated in Chapter 3. If a laboratory's CV only slightly exceeds the group CV, the probability for a single proficiency test result to exceed ± 2S limits is somewhat greater than 5%.

While fixed limits are easily implemented and can be related to medical usefulness requirements, their primary advantage over ± 2S limits is that acceptable laboratories are not penalized when group performance is much better than medical usefulness requirements.

In Table 11–4, the maximum efficiency of fixed limits is 93% and is not significantly better than that of ± 2S limits. At this efficiency, only 31% of the bad laboratories are identified due to the low prevalence of bad laboratories (10% or less). If the fundamental purpose of proficiency testing is to detect *bad* laboratories, the statistical and fixed limit approaches are both ineffective. Because both approaches pass good laboratories most of the time, current proficiency testing approaches are often mistaken for an effective program. This inability to correctly identify good and bad laboratories has serious ramifications as regulators increase their demands for documentation of acceptable intralaboratory performance.

Clearly, in the long term, alternative grading techniques must be developed to more accurately identify both good and bad intralaboratory performance.

USE OF GRADES

All proficiency testing programs provide the participant with comparisons of the laboratory's results to target values. These comparisons are usually in the form of "grades" based on the closeness of results to the target values. The grades are used for 2 purposes: (1) To determine passing or failing performance (by the regulator) and (2) To assess performance (by the participant).

Grades do not readily identify inferior performance. With large standard deviations or with large fixed limits, a very small fraction of bad laboratories are detected. As a result, the laboratory director or the regulatory agency, using the proficiency testing-grading process outlined above, may be lulled into a false sense of security, and may fail to note inadequate performance.

A failing grade should elicit considerable attention in the laboratory, and consistently failing grades should also elicit attention from the regulatory agency. A single failing grade amid consistently acceptable results is almost certainly indicative of a statistical outlier. Since most of the evaluation criteria are based on 95% confidence limits, approximately 1 in 20 proficiency testing results will exceed these limits even with acceptable performance. However, several failing results for one analyte, in which the errors are in the same direction, are indicative of either an analytical bias in the method, or a laboratory whose result is grouped in the wrong method.

Matrix effects (see above) can cause results to be placed in a wrong method group, ie, with a dissimilar set of chemical methodologies or instruments. For example, in some surveys a participant using a method which has fewer than 20 participants is graded against the grand mean, which may be heavily biased by an extremely popular method. For example, the Abbott TD_x method for digoxin was reported by over 50% of the participants in a recent CAP Survey; sparsely represented double-antibody RIA method users were graded in this survey against the grand mean, effectively the Abbott TD_x mean.

Laboratories often calibrate 2 or more methods or instruments within the laboratory to yield the same result on freshly collected patient specimens. Because of matrix effects, such a calibration scheme may cause otherwise reliable instruments to fail proficiency testing. For example, the Technicon SMAC chemistry analyzer, when calibrated to the Dupont ACA, will almost always fail proficiency testing when it is grouped with other SMACs, and paradoxically, when it is grouped with the ACAs. In this case, we would recommend that only the ACA proficiency test results be submitted for comparison to other ACAs, and that patient samples be used daily to verify the agreement of the ACA and SMAC.

Despite the inadequacies of the current grading schemes, grading will remain an integral part of proficiency testing programs. In the future, algorithms used for grading will be improved; it is anticipated that more effective rules will be utilized with better-defined criteria; ultimately, a multirule version of the approach may be incorporated. At present, use of proficiency testing grades should be a matter of utmost concern to the laboratory director. Any proposed grading system should not be implemented until its performance has been characterized by probability or simulation studies similar to those described above.

IMPACT OF UNETHICAL PARTICIPANT PRACTICES

It must be realized that passing or failing proficiency testing is not the definitive evaluation of intralaboratory performance. Whether proficiency testing programs use the traditional mean $\pm 2S$ criterion or fixed limits, regulators cannot guarantee adequate intralaboratory performance or provide the assurance that medical usefulness goals are being met. Both regulators and laboratory professionals must consider these shortcomings whenever interpreting proficiency testing results. The failure of proficiency testing to guarantee satisfactory intralaboratory performance does not detract from the ability of a laboratory to use proficiency testing to improve performance; it only reflects the inadequacy of proficiency testing as the report card.

Performance on proficiency surveys can be improved with simple practices, such as reanalyzing the proficiency specimens. Cembrowski and Vanderlinde found that a large proportion of Pennsylvania hospital laboratories perform multiple analyses of proficiency specimens and submit the means or median results.[25] The effect of analyzing the proficiency specimen several times and reporting the mean or median is clearly demonstrated by Table 11–2. If a laboratory's CV is 8%, and the specimen is analyzed 3 times, the CV of the mean is reduced to 5% and the probability of an unacceptable result is reduced from 20% to 5%! Not shown is the reduction of the survey S by this practice and the penalty to laboratories which treat the proficiency specimen as a patient specimen and analyze it only once. Boone et al used special

CDC surveys but were unable to demonstrate collusion among laboratories to obtain the "best" proficiency result.[26]

INFORMATION AVAILABLE TO PARTICIPANTS

The participant must be aware that the reported performance probably reflects the best that can be achieved. Cembrowski and Vanderlinde have reported that proficiency specimens are typically accorded special handling.[25] Human nature virtually assures that we strive more vigorously to do well when our results are reviewed.

Comparison to Peer Laboratories

The main benefit of proficiency testing is the ability to provide a rapid comparison to laboratories using equivalent methods and systems. A failure to provide comparable data is usually indicative of a large error in calibration. As laboratories acquire more instrument systems which are totally manufacturer "packaged," from instrumental design through exclusive reagent and calibration systems, the ability to improve the analytical performance decreases. Since some of these instruments can provide up to 60 different procedures, the laboratory becomes dependent on these instruments for particular analytes. In most cases, the laboratory has no inhouse basis for comparison—neither a method on a second instrument nor a secondary or backup method. As a result, the only assurances of adequate performance are obtained through the quality control information, where the possibility of a matrix effect in the value assignment process cannot be eliminated, or through inspection of the proficiency testing results. Because matrix effects cannot be excluded, the interlaboratory-intramethod comparisons (eg, DuPont ACAs in participating laboratories) check only for consistency. However, if the premise is accepted that the manufacturer is unbiased in calibration, proficiency testing is a valuable means of detecting atypical performance. Because proficiency testing programs are effective in detecting atypical performance, the further growth of voluntary, manufacturer-sponsored programs may be anticipated, particularly as professional programs become more regulatory in nature.

Comparative Methodology Performance

The interlaboratory coefficients of variation (CV) reported in proficiency testing programs are indirect measures of the intralaboratory CV which may be achieved by a particular method or instrument.

Because these interlaboratory CVs are due to calibration differences as well as intralaboratory (intrainstrument) variation, they will always exceed the intralaboratory CV. A comparison of the interlaboratory CVs provides the careful reviewer with a means of comparing operational characteristics of various analytical systems. This information is particularly helpful in the selection and purchase of an instrument and the evaluation of one's own intralaboratory performance.

DETERMINING BIAS

Ideally, proficiency testing results should be randomly distributed about the mean with equal numbers of positive and negative errors. A good estimate of the bias can be made from 10 or more samples. *Significant* bias is indicated in a proficiency testing program when all grades fall on the same side of the mean and deviate from the mean by more than $1S$. If significant bias exists, recalibration should be considered to bring the survey results closer to the group mean. As a first step, the laboratory should recalibrate the instrument according to manufacturer's directions and determine if the bias is corrected as measured by a group of samples (and possibly old survey specimens) analyzed before and after recalibration. As was shown in Chapter 6, the calibration process is imprecise, since a limited number of replicates of each calibrator are analyzed. If several calibrations are performed, the one which provides the change suggested by the survey results would be chosen. If the bias persists, new calibrators should be obtained from the manufacturer or another laboratory to verify or reject the previous calibration. If the bias persists, technical help should be sought from the manufacturer, colleagues, and other users. A cause for the bias should be uncovered. The practice of simply "tweaking" the method to bring the results onto the survey mean just obscures the problem and is not recommended.

MAXIMIZING TESTING BENEFITS

It is not necessary or even desirable to participate in every survey that is offered. Survey programs should be chosen carefully so that both the laboratory needs and regulatory/accreditation requirements are satisfied. In addition to the cost of the program, participation in a survey program is expensive in terms of time and materials. Some considerations for program selection follow:

1. Each area of testing should be covered by proficiency testing. Start

with the broadest groupings first (ie, general chemistry, immunoassay, toxicology, hematology, etc), then add the "specialty" surveys which focus on single analytes such as alcohol and CEA. Be sure sensitive analytes, such as those with increased legal ramifications, are well covered. Avoid analyte overlaps as much as possible in order to cover more analytes. Omit tests from surveys if they are well covered and better served by other surveys.

2. Take advantage of manufacturers' surveys whenever possible. These surveys generally provide educational benefits which are specific for method/instrument combinations, and the survey summaries can be extremely beneficial for self improvement.

3. Avoid surveys with excessive turnaround times.

4. Select surveys with thorough, intelligible, educational reports. Confusing or perfunctory reports will contribute little to performance improvement.

5. Select surveys in which your laboratory's methods will be part of a large homogeneous peer group. When there are only 1 to 5 participants reporting results from a particular method it is difficult to interpret survey results.

6. If you are uncomfortable about an analyte, use several different surveys in order to get more frequent comparative information and possibly another perspective.

CAP guidelines and Medicare/CLIA regulations require proficiency testing results be available and shared with bench level personnel. Such feedback maximizes the benefits of proficiency testing participation. The axiom "You get out of something what you put into it" applies to proficiency testing; especially if it is to be used as a part of a quality assurance program.

1. *Laboratory director*—The proficiency testing results are usually first received by the laboratory director who should scan them and focus on the bad grades. We advocate a policy whereby laboratory supervisors and/or bench level technologists performing tests are required to investigate causes for failing grades and to explain them in writing. Since most programs define 5% of the results to be outliers, isolated statistical outliers may be the most frequent explanation; however, followup of increased imprecision or significant bias is extremely important. The comments should be discussed at the monthly quality control review by the director and supervisor (see Chapter 12).

The director can help the supervisor develop a rational approach to the review of proficiency results and efficient problem-solving strategies. The director may be more able to recognize that a particular strategy is not working with a recurring problem and that a fresh approach is required. In the experience of the authors, repeated proficiency testing problems, despite extensive troubleshooting, recalibrations, and manufacturer's assistance, often indicate the need for method replacement. Such decisions are often initiated by the laboratory director.

The director should also take advantage of the opportunity to "point with pride" to good (passing) results. These should be acknowledged, in writing, usually on the report to the staff.

2. *Laboratory supervisor*—Interlaboratory survey programs are a valuable source of information, particularly when the laboratory is setting up a new test. In addition to verifying accuracy or demonstrating inaccuracy, surveys often provide "nuts and bolts" information about methodologies, interferences, and interpretation of patient test results. Supervisors should not limit their attention to failing results. All survey data should be reviewed carefully for trends and other information.

When failing results occur, the supervisor and analyst(s) should conduct an in-depth analysis of the proficiency testing data. They should first review the laboratory records for a clerical or calculation error and reconfirm specimen identification. The proficiency test results should be correlated to the routine quality control data produced over the same period that the proficiency test data were obtained.

If possible, survey materials should be retained for retesting, one of the most important phases of troubleshooting. When specimen contamination or a specimen reconstitution error is strongly suspected, it may be prudent to obtain and test new samples of the proficiency testing specimen. Acceptable results obtained upon retesting indicate analytical error during the initial testing period. If 2 or more specimen results were shifted in the same direction and reanalysis reveals no error, a transient bias was encountered. If there is no pattern in the initial proficiency results and reanalysis shows no error, then increased imprecision was previously encountered. A long-term bias is the most likely explanation when the retesting shows little difference between the 2 sets of proficiency results. In this case, calibration should be checked with specimen results verified by another method.

3. *Analyst*—Each analyst who has produced proficiency test results should initial the results on the final proficiency testing program report. Whenever a failing grade is investigated, the exercise should be carried

out jointly by the analyst and the supervisor in the spirit of learning. Rational explanations should be sought and accepted. Artefactual results, statistical outliers, and poor samples are examples of reasonable and acceptable explanations in the absence of information which demonstrates a problem.

4. *Laboratory staff*—The proficiency testing data, reports, and their explanations should be the subject of regular staff meetings, quality circles, or other departmental discussions. Solutions to problems should be sought; the merits of "explanations" should be evaluated and, where appropriate, accepted. Staff suggestions should be sought and considered before receipt of the next proficiency testing specimens. The staff should be made aware of the fallacies of proficiency testing—both good and bad grades must be interpreted with care and understanding. The role of proficiency testing in the laboratory quality assurance program must be carefully explained to staff members at all levels.

5. *Inspector*—The proficiency testing report, the notes added by the director, the supervisor, and the analysts, the explanations of "bad" grades, and the notes from the staff meeting where the results were discussed constitute a complete record which should be available to the inspector. This record provides all of the required information and demonstrates that the laboratory is maximizing the benefits of participation in the program.

6. *Outside the laboratory*—The laboratory should not hesitate to post excellent proficiency testing results on a bulletin board near the laboratory, along with a commendatory note from the director. Such a device will remind the nonlaboratory staff that quality work is being carried out. After all, most professional staff in other parts of the hospital/clinic do not undergo the rigorous outside inspections and proficiency testing programs common in the clinical laboratories.

OPPORTUNITIES

Proficiency testing is analogous to statistical quality control, and has some of the same limitations and shortcomings. One major difference is that outlying quality control results can be immediately investigated to solve a problem or demonstrate that a problem does not exist, whereas outlying proficiency results are investigated long after the fact. Another major difference is the statistical sample size; quality control results are available almost continuously, whereas proficiency results are supplied infrequently. Thus, far more is at stake with individual proficiency results, and there is so much pressure to perform acceptably that the results may no longer represent the usual testing process.

Increased use of multirule grading procedures with an attendant decrease in false rejections will improve proficiency testing. If a 1_{2s} rule violation is simply a warning in reference sample quality control, without consequence when it is an isolated event, it should be treated similarly in proficiency testing. The performance characteristics of the grading schemes commonly used in proficiency testing are just beginning to be understood, yet failure as defined by these schemes already has serious regulatory ramifications.

With the high prevalence of special handling and replicate testing of proficiency specimens, proficiency testing as it is currently practiced can provide a more reliable characterization of a laboratory's accuracy (bias) than its precision. In the future, proficiency testing programs could take advantage of these special practices, and require enough replicates on each sample so that a laboratory's bias can be measured accurately. With sufficient replicates, the laboratory's bias would become the dominant component of error of the mean, and a laboratory would be less able to provide a good appearance by merely running more replicates. Reliable estimates of precision are more difficult to develop; Kafka has used intralaboratory reference sample quality control data to assess precision in conjunction with interlaboratory proficiency testing.[27]

Proficiency testing, despite its limitations, can still achieve most of the benefits envisioned by its creators. The attitude of laboratory administration is critical; attitudes begin at the top. Although poor proficiency testing results should be a cause for concern, they should not be perceived as an indictment of poor laboratory performance. Rather, they should indicate the presence of an opportunity for improvement. Because the grading system is weak and can be defeated by relatively simple practices, skill is required to interpret proficiency testing results in the context of the whole laboratory quality assurance program. Proficiency testing's value as a regulatory tool is limited; its real value is to the sincere participant as a means of self-improvement.

REFERENCES

1. Belk WP, Sunderman FW: A survey of the accuracy of chemical analysis in clinical laboratories. Am J Clin Pathol 17:853-861, 1947.
2. Sunderman FW: The origin of proficiency testing for clinical laboratories in the United States. In: Proceedings of Second National Conference on Proficiency Testing. Information Services, Bethesda, Maryland, 1975, p 6.

3. Skendzel LP, Copeland BE: An international laboratory survey. Am J Clin Pathol 63:1007-1011, 1975.

4. Dorsey, DB: The evolution of proficiency testing in the USA. In Proceedings of Second National Conference on Proficiency Testing. Information Services, Bethesda, Maryland, 1975, pp 8-9.

5. Eilers RJ: Total quality control for the medical laboratory: the role of the College of American Pathologists Survey Program. Am J Clin Pathol 54:435-436, 1970.

6. U.S. Department of Health, Education and Welfare, Social Security Administration, 1968. Federal health insurance for the aged. Regulations for coverage of service of independent laboratories. DHEW Publ No. H1R-13.

7. U.S. Department of Health, Education and Welfare, Public Health Service, Centers for Disease Control, 1967. From Federal Register, vol 33, No. 253, December 31, 1968 (F.R. Doc. 68-155586).

8. Forney JE, et al: Laboratory evaluation and certification. In Inhorn SE, ed: Quality Assurance Practices for Health Laboratories. American Public Health Association, Washington, DC, 1977, pp 127-171.

9. Wilcox KR, et al: Laboratory management. In Inhorn SE, ed: Quality Assurance Practices for Health Laboratories. American Public Health Association, Washington, DC, 1977, pp 3-126.

10. Annino JS: What does laboratory "quality control" really control? N Engl J Med 299:1130, 1978.

11. Standards Committee, College of American Pathologists. Guideline for evaluating laboratory performance in survey and proficiency testing programs. Am J Clin Pathol 49:457-458, 1968.

12. Skendzel LP: Guidelines for the design of laboratory's surveys. Am J Clin Pathol 54:437-447, 1970.

13. Elevitch FR, Noce PS, eds: Data recap 1970–1980. College of American Pathologists, Skokie, Illinois, 1981.

14. Interlaboratory Comparison Program: CAP Surveys Manual, Section III, Chemistry. College of American Pathologists, Skokie, Illinois, 1987, pp 9-10.

15. Health Care Financing Administration, United States Government, Interpretive Guidelines for Independent Laboratories, Washington, DC, 1986.

16. Ehrmeyer SS, Laessig RH: Use of alternative rules (other than the 1_{2s}) for evaluating interlaboratory PT performance data. Clin Chem 34:250-256, 1988.

17. Gilbert RK, Platt R: The measurement of calcium and potassium in clinical laboratories in the United States, 1971-1978. Am J Clin Pathol 50:671-676, 1978.

18. Interlaboratory Comparison Program: CAP Surveys Manual, Section II, Hematology-Coagulation/Clinical Microscopy. College of American Pathologists, Skokie, Illinois, 1987, p 15.

19. Ehrmeyer SS, Laessig RH: An analysis of the use of the 1_{2s} rule to detect substandard performance in proficiency testing. Clin Chem 33:788-791, 1987.

20. Ehrmeyer SS, Laessig RH: An evaluation of proficiency testing programs' ability to determine intralaboratory performance: peer group statistics versus clinical usefulness limits. Arch Pathol Lab Med 112:444-448, 1988.

21. Ehrmeyer SS, Laessig RH: Alternative statistical approach to evaluating interlaboratory performance. Clin Chem 31:106-108, 1985.

22. Ehrmeyer SS, Laessig RH: Adequacy of interlaboratory precision criteria to measure intralaboratory performance. Clin Chem 31:1352-1354, 1983.

23. Ehrmeyer SS, Laessig RH: Interlaboratory proficiency testing programs: a computer model to assess their capability to correctly characterize intralaboratory performance. Clin Chem 33:784-787, 1987.

24. Ehrmeyer SS, Laessig RH: The effect of intralaboratory bias and imprecision on laboratories' ability to meet medical usefulness limits. Am J Clin Pathol 89:14-18, 1988.

25. Cembrowski GS, Vanderlinde R: Survey of special practices associated with College of American Pathologists proficiency testing in the Commonwealth of Pennsylvania. Arch Pathol Lab Med 112:374-376, 1988.

26. Boone J, Hearn T, Lewis S: Assessment of extent to which laboratories compare results before reporting in national laboratory performance surveys. Clin Chem 31:115, 1985.

27. Kafka MT: Internal quality control, proficiency testing and the clinical relevance of laboratory testing. Arch Pathol Lab Med 112:449-453, 1988.

28. Barnett RN: Medical significance of laboratory results. Am J Clin Pathol 50:671-676, 1968.

29. Skendzel LP, Barnett RN, Platt R: Medically useful criteria for analytic performance of laboratory tests. Am J Clin Pathol 83:200-205, 1985.

CHAPTER TWELVE

Requirements for Accreditation: Benefits to Quality Management

ACCREDITING AGENCIES

There is no single indicator that can be used by accrediting agencies to verify that a laboratory's total output meets the quality specifications for good patient care. Even very thorough audits of laboratory records and corresponding patient charts can be poor indicators of laboratory quality and can be fraught with interpretative biases. While proficiency testing results comprise the most readily available indicator of laboratory quality, Chapter 11 has shown that acceptable performance on proficiency testing does not rule out the presence of large, clinically important errors. Accrediting agencies seem to have recognized their inability to detect laboratory error, because their standards for accreditation emphasize prevention activities. On site accreditation inspections thus stress documentation of quality assurance and quality control activities rather than extensive auditing of laboratory and patient records.

Most hospital laboratories in the United States are accredited and inspected by either the College of American Pathologists (CAP) or the Joint Commission on Accreditation of Health Care Organizations (JCAHO). Some commercial laboratories receive accreditation from CAP. Both CAP and JCAHO publish standards which provide a framework for a laboratory's quality assurance program. As such, these standards are very important, and we have reproduced some of them as well as relevant portions of the CAP and JCAHO checklists, the series of detailed questions designed to implement the laboratory accreditation standards. These checklists are updated frequently; current versions are available from CAP or JCAHO. The materials presented below are summarized from checklists current in 1987 and 1989.

The standards for laboratory accreditation are continually evolving.

At its best, the spirit of the standards embodies the principles of quality management, and the standards provide an outline of a quality assurance program. At the least, the standards provide minimum benchmarks against which laboratories' quality practices can be judged. We have used some of these standards to introduce a discussion of the management role in quality assurance.

Quality Management Required by CAP

To receive and retain CAP accreditation the laboratory must satisfy CAP's basic Standards for Laboratory Accreditation. Standard III, Quality Assurance, states that

> "There shall be an ongoing quality assurance program designed to monitor and evaluate objectively and systematically the quality and appropriateness of the care and treatment provided to patients by the pathology service, to pursue opportunities to improve patient care, and to identify and resolve problems."[1]

Standard IV, which refers to quality control, states that

> "Each pathology service shall have a quality control system that demonstrates the reliability and medical usefulness of laboratory data."[1]

The interpretations which follow these 2 standards provide a list of components which make up the framework of a quality assurance program. They include

1. Responsibility of the laboratory director for the program of quality assurance.
2. Selection of test methods based on medical requirements.
3. Internal quality control system, clearly defined in writing, with evidence of understanding by laboratory personnel.
4. External quality control system.
5. Instrument maintenance program which monitors and demonstrates proper function of instruments.
6. Feedback mechanisms to assure medical usefulness of laboratory data.
7. Educational programs for personnel.
8. External audit or accreditation process.
9. Documentation of the above.
10. Procedure manuals in standard format, reviewed periodically.

249

11. Validation of methods before introduction and after out-of-control situations.

12. Specimen handling procedure manuals.

13. Surveillance and control of incoming materials (reagents and specimens).

While inspections by non-CAP organizations may be performed by a single individual, the CAP accrediting inspection is conducted by a team of peers from other CAP-accredited laboratories. These inspectors are encouraged to view themselves as "guest consultants."[2] The CAP inspection team verifies that the laboratory meets the CAP standards via a set of checklists of questions for each laboratory discipline. The CAP inspection process has the reputation of being more comprehensive than others because the inspection team is selected to have a broad range of laboratory skills. If necessary, a guest consultant will spend an entire day inspecting a single laboratory section. CAP inspectors are encouraged to adopt a positive attitude and to present observed deficiencies as recommendations for improvement.

The following examples are checklist questions dealing directly with quality control.[3] Each question is answered "yes," "no," or "N/A" (nonapplicable) by the inspector.

1. "Is the laboratory enrolled in a CAP survey (interlaboratory comparison) program appropriate for the testing performed?

2. "Is there evidence of active review by the pathologist or designated supervisor(s) of the survey results?

3. "Is there evidence of evaluation and, if indicated, corrective action in response to 'unacceptable' results on the survey report?" (Interpretation given for Standard IV requires that laboratory director and supervisory person record findings of investigation and corrective action and sign report.[1])

4. "Is there evidence of active review of results of controls, instrument maintenance and function, temperature, etc, for routine procedures on all shifts?

5. "Is there documentation of corrective action taken when controls, etc, exceed defined tolerance limits?

6. "Are control specimens at more than one level (normal and abnormal) used for all tests (when available)?

7. "Are tolerance limits defined for control procedures?"

Individual checklists are provided for hematology, chemistry, urinalysis, microbiology, blood bank, diagnostic immunology, histocompatability, laboratory general, and the limited service laboratory. In the area of clinical chemistry, there are separate checklists with specific quality control requirements for radioimmunoassay (nuclear medicine) and toxicology and therapeutic monitoring.

Quality Management Required by JCAHO

The approach of the JCAHO in accrediting basic quality control is similar to that of the CAP. The excerpts below are from the *Accreditation Manual for Hospitals, 1989*, copyright 1989 by the Joint Commission on Accreditation of Healthcare Organizations, Chicago, and are reprinted with permission. Standard PA.5 states

"Quality-control systems and measures of the pathology and medical laboratory services are designed to assure the medical reliability of laboratory data."[4]

Some of the characteristics directly related to quality control that are required of the laboratory are listed below.[4] Compliance with each characteristic is rated by the inspector on a scale of 1 (substantial compliance) to 5 (noncompliance).

1. "There is a documented quality-control program in effect for each section of the pathology and medical laboratory services.
2. "General quality controls required of and practiced by the pathology and medical laboratory service include, but need not be limited to, the following:
    a. "Use of proficiency testing programs for each discipline offered by the clinical laboratory.
    b. "There is a complete written description of each test procedure, including control and calibration procedures and pertinent literature references.
    c. "Documentation of remedial action taken for detected deficiencies/defects identified through quality-control measures or authorized inspections.
    d. "Quality control records are retained for at least two years.
3. For clinical chemistry specifically:
    a. "Each procedure in clinical chemistry is verified by appropriate controls at least once on each day of use.
    b. "Data are available to document the routine precision of test results and the schedule of recalibration.
    c. "At least one standard and one reference sample are included with each run of unknown specimens when such standards and reference samples are available.
    d. "Standard deviation, coefficient of variation, or other statis-

251

tical estimates are determined by random replicate testing of specimens.

e. "Acceptable limits for all standard and reference quality-control samples are established and are available to laboratory personnel, as is the course of action to be instituted when results are outside the satisfactory control limits.

f. "Control limits on all tests are established to produce results commensurate with meaningful clinical applications."

Standard PA.7 expands the JCAHO approach further into quality management, stating

"As part of the hospital's quality assurance program, the quality and appropriateness of pathology and medical services are monitored and evaluated, and identified problems are resolved."

The characteristics required to meet this standard are more clinically oriented, and generally similar to the characteristics of quality management described in Chapter 1; some of them are

a. "The quality and appropriateness of patient care services are monitored and evaluated in all major functions of the pathology and medical laboratory department/service.

b. "Such monitoring and evaluation are accomplished through the following means:
   1. "Routine collection in the pathology and medical laboratory department/service, or through the hospital's quality assurance program, of information about important aspects of pathology and medical laboratory services; and
   2. "Periodic assessment by the pathology and medical laboratory department/service of the collected information in order to identify important problems in patient care services and opportunities to improve care.
      (a). "In (#1 & #2, above) the pathology and medical laboratory department/service agrees on objective criteria that reflect current knowledge and clinical experience.
      (b). "These criteria are used by the pathology and medical laboratory/service, and other clinical departments/services as appropriate, or by the hospital's quality assurance program in the monitoring and evaluation of patient care services.

c. "When important problems in patient care services or opportunities to improve care are identified, actions are taken; and the effectiveness of the actions taken is evaluated.

d. "As part of the annual reappraisal of the hospital's quality assurance program, the effectiveness of the monitoring, evaluation, and problem-solving activities in the pathology and medical laboratory department/service is evaluated."

HCFA Requirements

Most independent laboratories (commercial laboratories) which are approved for Medicare testing in the United States must meet the requirements of the federal government's Health Care Financing Administration (HCFA). The HCFA guidelines and inspection checklist[5] cover most of the issues covered in the CAP inspection checklist; the HCFA guidelines are more specific and leave less to interpretation. They are legal regulations defining minimum standards for laboratory operation.

Generally HCFA guidelines set minimum standards on some very specific issues; for example, HCFA guidelines specify that at least 1 calibrator and 1 control must be included with each run of unknown specimens except:

1. If calibrators are not used, 2 controls of different concentrations must be used.
2. If controls are not used, 2 calibrators of different concentrations must be used.
3. A calibrator and a sample spiked with calibrator may be used.
4. For analyzers with prepackaged reagents, for each test, a standard at the upper limit of the reportable range and a control within the normal range must be run once per day.

Other areas in which the guidelines are very specific include

1. Number of standards required for calibration of different methods.
2. Criteria for determining the acceptability of proficiency test results.
3. Approved proficiency testing programs and minimum requirements for proficiency testing program approval.

HCFA guidelines, as those of the CAP and JCAHO, do not define specific tolerance limits for interpretation of quality control results. For all 3 organizations, the individual laboratory must specify the tolerance limits; however, they all require documentation of appropriate responses to recognized out-of-control situations.

DOCUMENTATION

Clearly, documentation is one of the most important requirements for accreditation, as well as for a successful quality control program.

253

Each analytical procedure must be totally specified; the quality control procedure is an important part of this specification. In our experience, the quality control system is most susceptible to breakdown at the control results interpretation step. If the quality control procedure is not explicitly defined, interpretation of control data will be left to the discretion of the individual performing the test or checking the run.

Documentation alone is not sufficient; training alone is not sufficient. Supervisory personnel must set a clear example: they must be involved in the daily review of quality control data, especially when new employees are involved. Supervisory personnel must make clear which decisions are management's and which may be made by bench personnel. Teaching by example is very important, as many view quality control as a highly abstract process.

When control data violate quality control rules, the decision to accept or reject the run must be documented. Even if the violation is a "warning," it should be duly noted. Suspected or actual causes of control problems should be documented. All corrective actions should be recorded. Documentation of previous run experiences will aid in the interpretation of subsequent control data and serves more than just satisfying accreditation and legal requirements.

The standardized treatment of control data will yield statistically valid control limits. If only warning rules are violated, the control results must be retained for statistical calculations. Otherwise, the ranges will become too narrow. Documentation of the responses to control rule violations can check the tendency to repeat warnings and to report only the good results

SUPERVISORY REVIEW

Runs whose results fail quality control rules should be brought to the attention of the supervisor or designated checker. When combination rules are used, and the false rejection rate is low, effort should be directed to determine the cause of the failure and to correct it before the run is repeated. As pointed out previously, an error must be very large before it can be consistently detected by combination rules.

On a regular basis, perhaps weekly, all failed and warning runs should be reviewed to determine the presence of significant systematic or random error. Such review is especially important when computerized quality control systems are used and control data are not plotted daily. Retrospective analysis rules may be helpful in detecting these trends (see Multistage Control Procedures, Chapter 8).

Control problems which have not been adequately handled should immediately be brought to the attention of the involved personnel. Over a period as short as several days, the circumstances of a control decision can be forgotten, and reminders about quality control procedures become abstract.

At monthly intervals, all control data should be examined for possible trends, preferably in graphical format, by the supervisor or responsible person. Other data, such as temperature monitoring, spectrophotometer checks, etc, should also be reviewed for trends and compliance with monitoring procedures. A summary report should be prepared which integrates the problems detected, corrective actions, and interpretations of the proficiency test results received that month.

TOP MANAGEMENT'S ROLE

The laboratory director has ultimate responsibility for all quality management activities in the laboratory. To be maximally effective, the director should be actively involved in the administration of the laboratory. The CAP checklist for "Laboratory General" asks,

> "Is there evidence that the Laboratory Director has sufficient authority to influence the quality of medical patient services by decisions relative to the selection of methods, equipment and personnel; and is actively involved in the daily affairs of the laboratory?"[6]

> "Is the Laboratory Director actively involved in the daily affairs and the quality control of the laboratory?"

Consistent achievement of quality can occur only if top management is totally committed to quality management. Townsend in *Commit to Quality*[7] terms the corporation's chief executive officer (CEO) the "indispensable participant." In the laboratory the indispensable participant is the laboratory director. The director must have a detailed understanding of the operation of the quality assurance program at all levels, and be committed to carry out the program if subordinates fail. Subordinates will judge the extent of the commitment to quality by the director's actions. The director sets the tone or the attitude of the staff and therefore must exemplify a compassionate standard of patient care. The director's role includes representing the quality management interests of the laboratory to (the hospital's) top management; the credibility with top management will reflect the director's example.

Each section's monthly quality control summary should be reviewed jointly by the laboratory director and the appropriate section supervisor. The director will become more aware of problems encountered during the month and will be better able to assist in developing problem-solving strategies and providing appropriate clinical input. The director must delegate some quality management responsibilities to laboratory management and provide the opportunity for laboratory management to carry out these responsibilities. Because formal training in quality assurance has generally been weak, the director and supervisors must often serve as quality assurance tutors. This further underscores the importance of management's role in setting the right example.

Either unilaterally or in conjunction with the hospital's quality assurance organization (and other appropriate organizations), laboratory management establishes the quality assurance program of the laboratory. They first determine which quality characteristics of the laboratory should be monitored. They then determine the performance standards, set up monitoring procedures, interpret the incoming data, and determine whether corrective actions are necessary.

A typical example of these quality management activities, introduced in Chapter 1, involves evaluating the turnaround time for routine morning testing on specimens from patients in high-intensity nursing units. In conjunction with the medical staff at one of our hospitals, we established a standard of delivering computer printouts of the routine morning test results to the nursing stations before 9 AM at least 90% of the time (the laboratory is responsible for morning phlebotomy). The times at which the routine testing is finished in the Chemistry and Hematology laboratories and the times at which the reports leave the laboratory are monitored manually. The times when individual specimens arrive in the laboratory and the times when each test is completed are monitored by computer, and summary reports of these times are generated by the computer. When the performance standard is not met for reasons other than equipment failure, delayed specimens are investigated to discover common sources of delay. Corrective actions have included correcting instrument service problems, increasing service training of laboratory personnel, improving specimen handling and testing processes, and increasing the laboratory personnel's awareness of the need for rapid turnaround time. The immediate benefit of this program has been that we are actively controlling quality in a quantitative sense. A side benefit is that the laboratory no longer falls prey to anecdotal statements by Emergency Department staff about how long the lab takes to do a test; both parties know that the laboratory is monitoring and controlling turnaround time.

THE ROLE OF LABORATORY PERSONNEL

The emphasis placed on management's role is not meant to minimize the role of the laboratory employees in achieving quality. Everyone must be involved and committed to achieving quality. The bench level personnel must continually be challenged to provide their ideas for improvement. As the old saying goes, "If you really want to know what's going on, ask the person doing the work." There are many aspects of the laboratory with which bench level personnel are much more familiar than management—after all, they observe the problems every day. They know which methods are not working well, often before management recognizes a problem via the control data or erroneous patient data.

Laboratory personnel are highly motivated toward producing quality work. This motivation becomes very apparent with a little encouragement and example-setting, even if formal training in quality assurance and quality control may have been limited. Bench level personnel must be involved in the quality improvement process, not only in their usual testing role, but also as a source of ideas on how to improve the testing process.

REFERENCES

1. College of American Pathologists, Standards for laboratory accreditation, Commission on Laboratory Accreditation. Skokie, Illinois, 1987.

2. College of American Pathologists, Inspector's manual for accreditation of medical laboratories, Commission on Laboratory Accreditation. Skokie, Illinois, 1980.

3. College of American Pathologists, Clinical chemistry inspection checklist, Commission on Laboratory Accreditation. Skokie, Illinois, 1987.

4. Joint Commission on Accreditation of Health Care Organizations, Accreditation manual for hospitals, Chicago, 1985.

5. Health Care Financing Administration, United States Government, Interpretive Guidelines for Independent Laboratories, Washington, DC, October, 1986.

6. College of American Pathologists, Laboratory general inspection checklist, Commission on Laboratory Accreditation, Skokie, Illinois, 1987.

7. Townsend PL: Commit to Quality. John Wiley & Sons, New York, 1986.

Index

Numbers in *italic* refer to pages on which illustrations or tables appear.

Smoothing constant, 26–28, *27, 52–53,
55*
Smoothing mean, *156*
Specimen
 sample, 230–31
 sample mixups, 144–45, *145,* 146
Standard deviation, 13–14, *14,* 17, 97
 between day, 19–20
 between run, 19–20
 calculation of, *15*
 of the duplicates, 14
 of the mean (SEM), 16
 of the observations, 27–28
 within lot, 103–4
 within run, 18–19
 total, 20
Standard deviation index (SDI), 14, *14,*
 231
 ±2S limits, 234, *235*
Standard error of the mean (SEM), 16
Startup quality control, 1
Statistics
 calculation of population, *15*
 population descriptions, 11–16, *12,
 14–15*
Systematic error (SE), 24, *25, 26, 35–36*

T

Technicon
 H1, 203
 SMAC, 238–39
Testing
 analytical stage of, 6–8, *7*
 and errors, 4–5
 internal/external, 8–9
 manufacturer, 229, 242
 maximizing benefits of, 241–44
 patient data and, 134–38
 of quality assurance, control, 5–6, *6,
 9*
 significance, 20–22, *21*
 steps for, quality, *3*
Timeliness, 3
Trend analysis, 50–52, *70*
 accuracy, 68
 precision, 53–54, 68

Truncation limits, 151, 152–53, *153*
T-test, 20–21, *21*
Turnaround times, 2–4, 230

V

Values
 predictive, 71–75, *72–74*
Variance, 13
 analysis of. *See* Analysis of variance
 analyst to analyst, 109
 between-run components of, 100–22
 biological, inherent, 22–23, *24*
 calculation example for, *15*
 calibration, 109–10
 of control materials, 108–9
 impact of between-run components
 on quality control procedures,
 111–22
 intraindividual, 22–23, *24*
 interindividual, 22–23, *24*
 long-term, *18,* 19–20
 physiological, 85–90
 reagent, 109
 short-term between-run components
 of, 106–8, *107*
 short-term within run, *18,* 18–19
 week-to-week, *18*
 within run, 18

W

Westgard multirule, 72, 75, 116–17, 179,
 183
White cell differential counts, 205–7, *206*
Within run variation, *18,* 18–19

X

$\bar{X}_{Pfr}$, 48–50, *50*
$\bar{X}$. *See* Mean
$\bar{X}_{0.01}$, *34*

Z

Z-score, 14, 49. *See also* Standard deviation index